PRACTICAL MANUAL
Of
NUTRITION AND DIETETICS

Dedicated to

to my family
and
dearest friends

PRACTICAL MANUAL Of NUTRITION AND DIETETICS

FIRST EDITION

PART - I	PART - II	PART - III
BASIC NUTRITION	NUTRITION FOR LIFESPAN	THERAPEUTIC NUTRITION
DR. AKANKSHA YADAV	DR. MONIKA ARORA	MS. SWAYAM SIDDHA

KALPAZ

First Published, 2019

Published by
Kalpaz Publications
C-30, Satyawati Nagar,
Delhi – 110052
E-mail: kalpaz@hotmail.com
Ph.: 9212142040

Printed at: G. Print Process, Delhi

Cataloging in Publication Data—DK
Courtesy: D.K. Agencies (P) Ltd. <docinfo@dkagencies.com>

Yadav, Akanksha, author.
Practical manual of nutrition and dietetics. — First edition.
pages cm
Includes bibliographical references.
Contents: part I. Basic nutrition / Dr. Akanksha Yadav — part II. Nutrition for lifespan / Dr. Monika Arora — part III. Therapeutic nutrition / Ms. Swayam Siddha.
ISBN 9789353240028

1. Nutrition. 2. Diet therapy. I. Arora, Monika (Writer on nutrition), author. II. Siddha, Swayam, author. III. Title.

LCC RA784.Y33 2019 | DDC 613.2 23

CONTENTS

PART III - THERAPEUTIC NUTRITION

ACKNOWLEDGEMENTS

First of all, we would like to thank almighty for blessing us to write this Nutrition Manual.

We express our heartfelt gratitude and respect to our families for their timely guidance, support and motivation to move forward.

One of the authors, Ms. Swayam Siddha, would like to extend thanks to her greatest inspiration Dr. Sarita Sachdeva, Dean, Faculty of Applied Science, Manav Rachna International Institute of Research and Studies and Dr V.K.Govilla, Dean, Faculty of Allied Health Sciences, SGT University for true support, motivation and for giving their valuable inputs.

Writing this manual is never an easy task. The inspiration of students motivated us to create a manual which will be helpful for teachers and students.

Our sincere thanks to Mr. B.P.Garg, Director, Gyan Book Publisher (P) Ltd who showed his trust and accepted the manuscript for publication.

Last but not the least the authors wants to thanks their colleagues and friends for their undue blessings and support and our respected teachers for imparting us the knowledge of the fundamental concepts in Nutrition sciences.

PREFACE

The workbook (manual) is directed primarily for the students of Nutrition & Dietetics, Food Science, Food technology, Nursing, Optometric technicians and a related subject up to Undergraduate's level and assumes some knowledge of basic nutrition. As nutrition professionals, we have reached this basic conclusion that practical part is more important than theory part. Theories will you give an idea but practically when you are doing the task/ activity you are learning through Gyanendriya.

Gyanendriya are the organs by which knowledge is acquired i.e. sense of sight, sense of smell, sense of hearing, sense of touch and sense of taste. Practically students not even learn but also experience through all sense organs and that experience is long lasting. These sense organs connected with these sense that take in information that is sent to the brain so that the body can act on it. We believe that through the practical process student will learn how to perform this activity as they are not gathering information not only through reading. This Manual is published with an ambitious aim to provide the students with a comprehensive practical knowledge. This book makes an attempt to inform and guide the students to learn on how to use the principles of Nutrition & Dietetics required for fulfilling the nutritional requirement of people at different stages of life. The first edition of practical manual consists of 36 exercises arranged into 3parts covering the following subjects:

PART ONE Basic Nutrition introduces the students the proper use and care of different types of kitchen equipments used in the nutrition laboratory, nutrition labelling and sources of different nutrients.

PART TWO Nutrition for Life Span acquaints students with proper use of exchange list in planning and preparation of a balanced diet for all vulnerable groups.

PART THREE Therapeutic Nutrition presents the standardization of food products and planning and preparation of therapeutic diets.

The format of each exercise in this workbook (manual) is intended to promote learning in the shortest possible time. Record the practical work directly into the bound practical manual (workbook), never on loose-leaf sheets. Every entry in the practical manual should be dated, and your own observations (including comments such as the difficulties you found in doing certain procedures, or ideas that occurred to you) should be written down as a permanent record. Recognize that your practical manual is the true record of what you did and observed at the time. You can (if you wish) use the back pages of your practical manual for making calculations, notes, etc. It's an attempt to simplify the work of both teachers and students as will provide all necessary information in a sequential manner with practical guidelines. We have included annexure (references) that we consider are among the most current at the time of writing, but have also taken the liberty of including some of the older, which we feel are well worth. We earnestly hope that students will enjoy reading, learning from the manual and also benefit from it as well as spread the valuable information among those around them.

PART - I

BASIC NUTRITION

DR. AKANKSHA YADAV

PRACTICAL NO. 1

USE AND CARE OF KITCHEN EQUIPMENTS

Aim:- To identify and enlist the use and care of different kitchen equipments used for preparation & cooking of food.

Sl. No.		*Name of Equipment*	*Types of Equipment*	*Use of Equipment*	*Care of Equipment*
1.	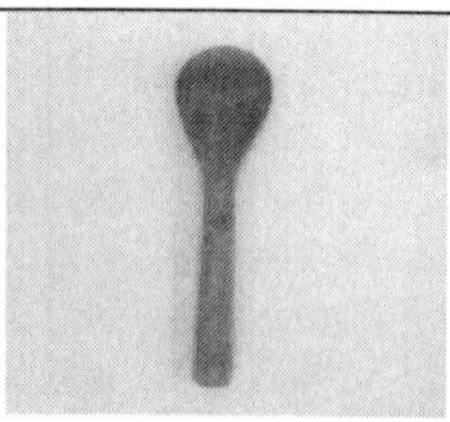				
2.	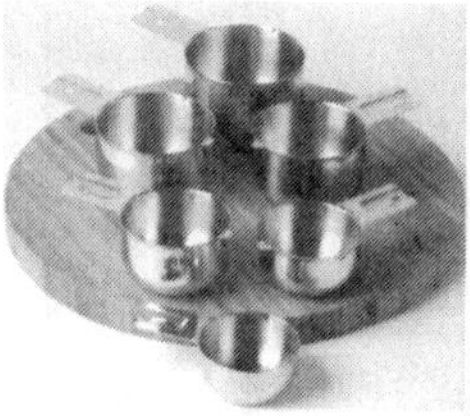				
3.	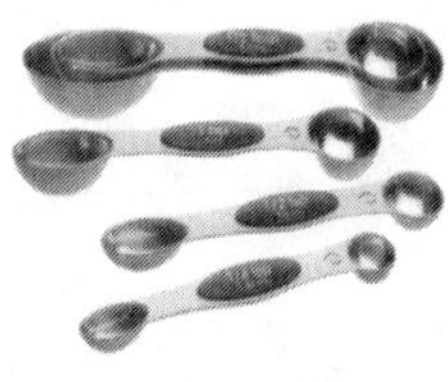				

4.	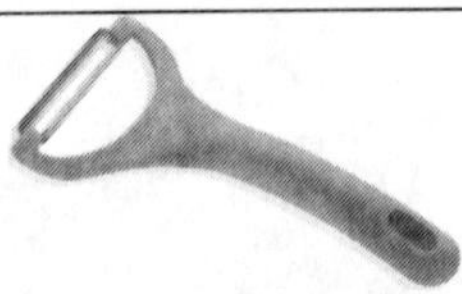				
5.	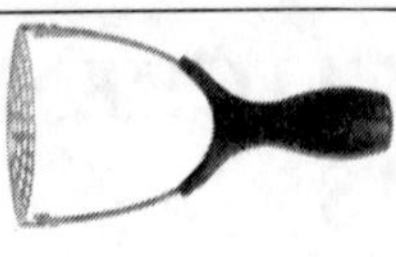				
6.	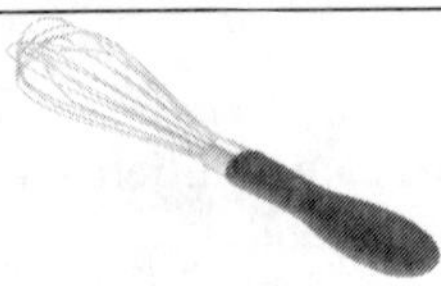				
7.	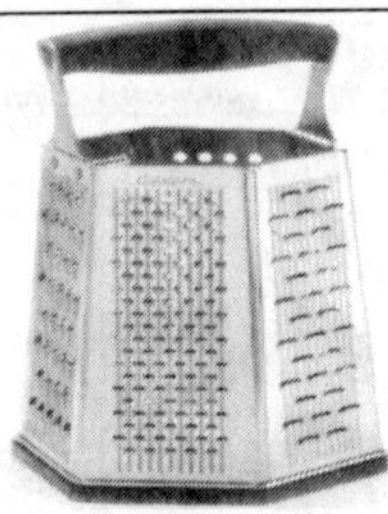				
8.	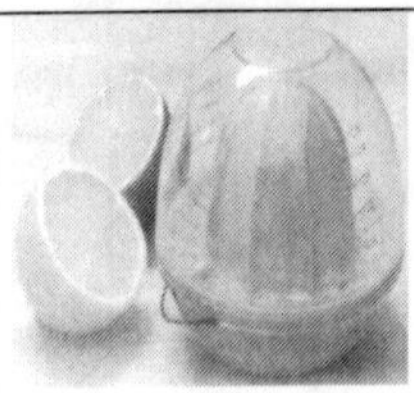				
9.	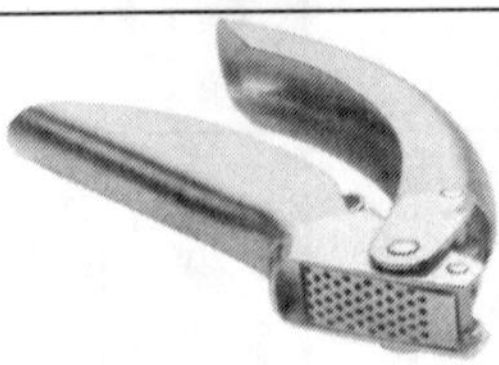				

10.	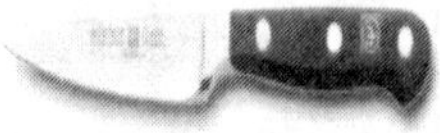				
11.	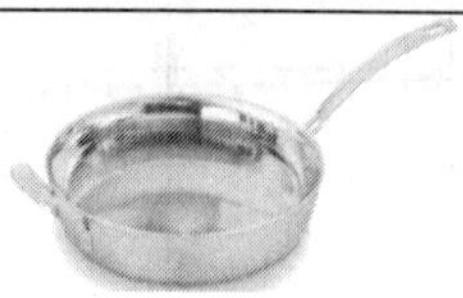				
12.	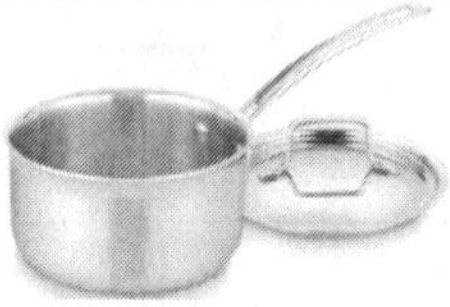				
13.	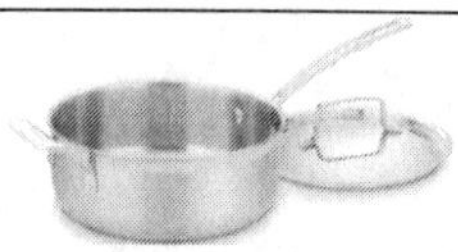				
14.	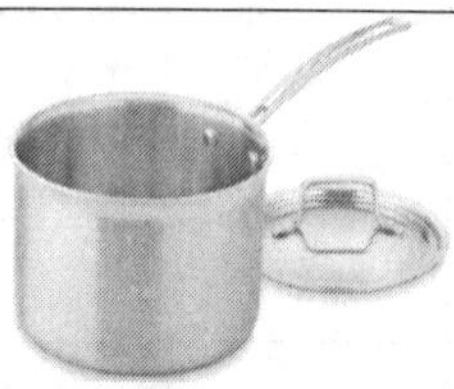				
15.	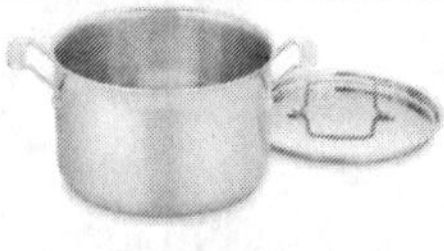				
16.	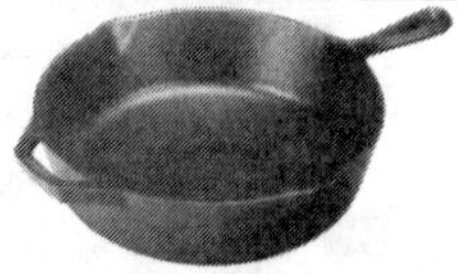				
17.	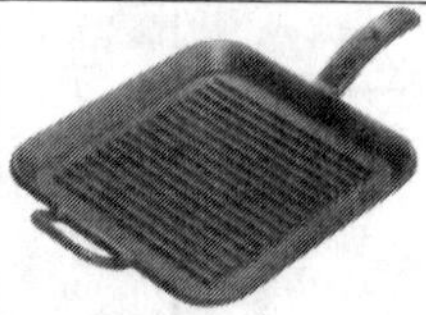				

18.	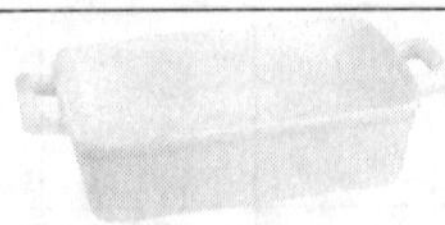		
19.	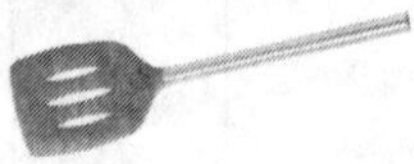		
20.	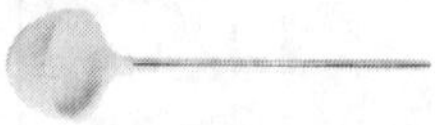		
21.	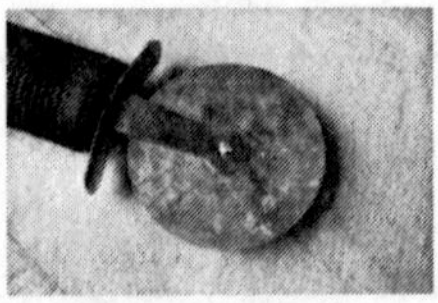		
22.	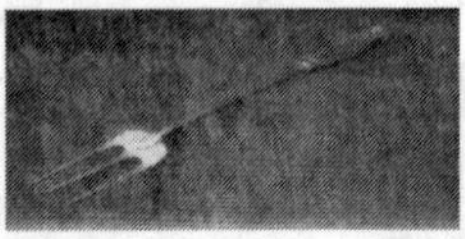		
23.	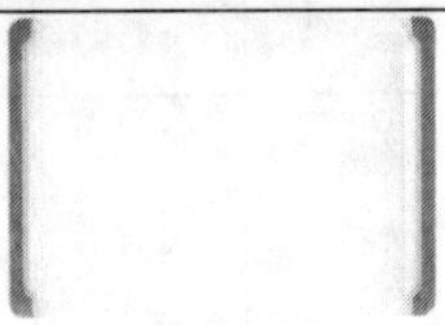		
24.	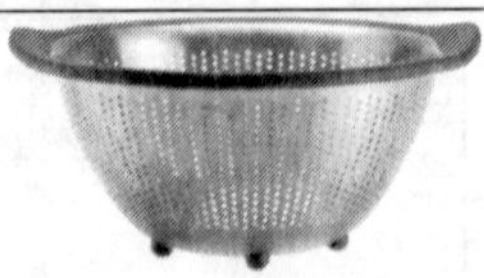		
25.	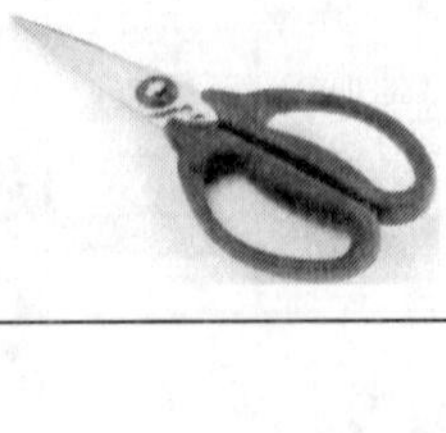		

26.					
27.	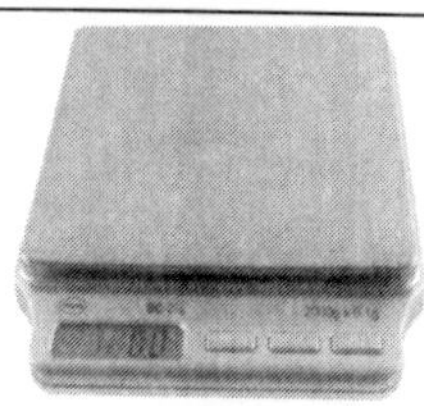				
28.	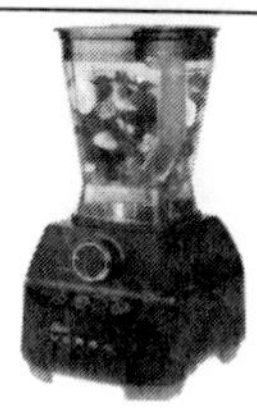				

Teachers Signature

PRACTICAL NO. 2

FOOD SOURCES OF NUTRIENTS

Aim: - To Enlist the sources of foods rich in nutrients- Energy, protein, Fats, Vitamins and Minerals. Calculate the nutritive value of per 100g of food with serving size

Mention at least 5 functions of each nutrient

SOURCES AND FUNCTIONS OF MACRONUTRIENTS

ENERGY

Sources	Kcal Per 100g	Serving Size(g)	Kcal per serving

FUNCTIONS:	DEFICIENCY	TOXICITY

PROTEIN

Sources	Kcal Per 100g	Serving Size(g)	Kcal per serving

FUNCTIONS:	DEFICIENCY	TOXICITY

FATS

Sources	Kcal Per 100g	Serving Size(g)	Kcal per serving

FUNCTIONS:	DEFICIENCY	TOXICITY

VITAMIN A

Sources	µg per 100g		Serving Size(g)	µg per serving
	Retinol	Carotene		

FUNCTIONS:	DEFICIENCY	TOXICITY

VITAMIN D

Sources	µg Per 100g	International Unit	Serving Size(g)	µg per serving

FUNCTIONS:	DEFICIENCY	TOXICITY

VITAMIN E

Sources	µg Per 100g	Serving Size(g)	µg per serving

FUNCTIONS:	DEFICIENCY	TOXICITY

VITAMIN K

Sources	µg Per 100g	Serving Size(g)	µg per serving

FUNCTIONS:	DEFICIENCY	TOXICITY

THAIMINE

Sources	Mg Per 100g	Serving Size(mg)	Mg per serving

FUNCTIONS:	DEFICIENCY	TOXICITY

FOLIC ACID

Sources	Mg Per 100g	Serving Size(mg)	Mg per serving

FUNCTIONS:	DEFICIENCY	TOXICITY

VITAMIN C

Sources	Mg Per 100g	Serving Size(mg)	Mg per serving

FUNCTIONS:	DEFICIENCY	TOXICITY

POTASSIUM

Sources	Mg Per 100g	Serving Size(mg)	Mg per serving

FUNCTIONS:	DEFICIENCY	TOXICITY

SODIUM

Sources	Mg Per 100g	Serving Size(mg)	Mg per serving

FUNCTIONS:	DEFICIENCY	TOXICITY

SULPHUR

Sources	Mg Per 100g	Serving Size(mg)	Mg per serving

FUNCTIONS:	DEFICIENCY	TOXICITY

SELENIUM

Sources	Mg Per 100g	Serving Size(mg)	Mg per serving

FUNCTIONS:	DEFICIENCY	TOXICITY

IRON

Sources	Mg Per 100g	Serving Size(mg)	Mg per serving

FUNCTIONS:	DEFICIENCY	TOXICITY

CALCIUM

Sources	Mg Per 100g	Serving Size(mg)	Mg per serving

FUNCTIONS:	DEFICIENCY	TOXICITY

ZINC

Sources	Mg Per 100g	Serving Size(mg)	Mg per serving

FUNCTIONS:	DEFICIENCY	TOXICITY

FIBRE

Sources	Soluble Fibre (gm per 100 gm of food)	Insoluble Fibre (gm per 100 gm of food)	Total Fibre (gm per 100 gm of food)

FUNCTIONS:	DEFICIENCY	TOXICITY

EXERCISE 1

Answer the following questions

Q1. Define Macronutrient and Micronutrient

Q2. Mention the amount of energy yielded by the following nutrient in a human body?

1 gm of Carbohydrate:

1 gm of Proteins:

1 gm of Fats:

1 gm of Alcohol:

Q3. Define Energy and unit of Energy

Q4. Discuss the importance of water in daily life

Q5. Define Nutrition & Dietetics and role of nutrition in day to day life

Teachers Signature

PRACTICAL NO. 3

PRICE LIST OF SEASONAL AVAILABLE FOOD

Aim:- To conduct the survey and make the list of prices of foods available throughout the year with their nutritional benefits

Note:- Make the list of food under different food groups and mention the particular season wherever required

PRICE LIST OF FOODS

Food Item	Location	Month	Price (Rs.) (ltr or kg)	Season	Nutritional Benefit
Milk & Milk Product					

Food Item	Location	Month	Price (Rs.) (in kg)	Season	Nutritional Benefit
Meat & Meat Products					
Pulses					

Food Item	Location	Month	Price (Rs.) (in kg)	Season	Nutritional Benefit
Cereals and cereal Products					
Green Leafy Vegetables					

Food Item	Location	Month	Price (Rs.) (in kg)	Season	Nutritional Benefit
Roots & Tubers					
Other Vegetables					
Fruits					

Food Item	Location	Month	Price (Rs.) (ltr or kg)	Season	Nutritional Benefit
Fats and Oils, Dry fruits					
Sugars					

EXERCISE 1

Q1. Enlist the Nutritious food items that can be given as a substitute to a lower Income Group to fulfil their nutritional requirement

Teachers Signature

PRACTICAL NO. 4

NUTRITIONAL LABELLING

Aim: - To conduct a Survey in a local market and prepare a list of different food products according to their nutrition label

General Information

In today's time lots of processed and raw food materials are manufactured by different food companies. Each product have a nutrition label which mentions the name of the manufacturing company, date of manufacturing date of expiry and the rate at which that particular product is available.

It is very essential that before buying any food item one should know the information given on the label very carefully. The nutritional label not only gives the information about the manufacturing but also gives the details about the nutritional value that product contains as well as the ingredients used in the production of that product

A good customer is the one who is aware of mislabelling and always read the label carefully before purchasing any processed or raw food product.

Write the detailed information provided on the nutrition label for the following products

INFORMATION ON NUTRITION LABEL

Labels	Milk & Milk Product		
Name of the product			
Net Weight			
Price			
Date of manufacturing			
Date of expiry			
Product code			
Serving size			
Nutritive value per 100g Energy Protein Fat MUFA PUFA Trans Fat Sugar			
Preservative added			
Ingredients			
Red Mark/ Green Mark			

Labels	**Meat & Meat Product**		
Name of the product			
Net Weight			
Price			
Date of manufacturing			
Date of expiry			
Product code			
Serving size			
Nutritive value per 100g Energy Protein Fat MUFA PUFA Trans Fat Sugar			
Preservative added			
Ingredients			
Red Mark/ Green Mark			

Labels	Pulses		
Name of the product			
Net Weight			
Price			
Date of manufacturing			
Date of expiry			
Product code			
Serving size			
Nutritive value per 100g Energy Protein Fat MUFA PUFA Trans Fat Sugar			
Preservative added			
Ingredients			
Red Mark/Green Mark			

Labels	Cereals		
Name of the product			
Net Weight			
Price			
Date of manufacturing			
Date of expiry			
Product code			
Serving size			
Nutritive value per 100g Energy Protein Fat MUFA PUFA Trans Fat Sugar			
Preservative added			
Ingredients			
Red Mark/Green Mark			

Labels	**Vegetables**		
Name of the product			
Net Weight			
Price			
Date of manufacturing			
Date of expiry			
Product code			
Serving size			
Nutritive value per 100g Energy Protein Fat MUFA PUFA Trans Fat Sugar			
Preservative added			
Ingredients			
Red Mark/Green Mark			

Labels	Fruits		
Name of the product			
Net Weight			
Price			
Date of manufacturing			
Date of expiry			
Product code			
Serving size			
Nutritive value per 100g Energy Protein Fat MUFA PUFA Trans Fat Sugar			
Preservative added			
Ingredients			
Red Mark/Green Mark			

Labels	Fats & Oils		
Name of the product			
Net Weight			
Price			
Date of manufacturing			
Date of expiry			
Product code			
Serving size			
Nutritive value per 100g Energy Protein Fat MUFA PUFA Trans Fat Sugar			
Preservative added			
Ingredients			
Red Mark/Green Mark			

Labels	Dry Fruits		
Name of the product			
Net Weight			
Price			
Date of manufacturing			
Date of expiry			
Product code			
Serving size			
Nutritive value per 100g Energy Protein Fat MUFA PUFA Trans Fat Sugar			
Preservative added			
Ingredients			
Red Mark/Green Mark			

Labels	Sugars		
Name of the product			
Net Weight			
Price			
Date of manufacturing			
Date of expiry			
Product code			
Serving size			
Nutritive value per 100g Energy Protein Fat MUFA PUFA Trans Fat Sugar			
Preservative added			
Ingredients			
Red Mark/Green Mark			

Labels	Functional Food		
Name of the product			
Net Weight			
Price			
Date of manufacturing			
Date of expiry			
Product code			
Serving size			
Nutritive value per 100g Energy Protein Fat MUFA PUFA Trans Fat Sugar			
Preservative added			
Ingredients			
Red Mark/Green Mark			

Labels	Organic Foods		
Name of the product			
Net Weight			
Price			
Date of manufacturing			
Date of expiry			
Product code			
Serving size			
Nutritive value per 100g Energy Protein Fat MUFA PUFA Trans Fat Sugar			
Preservative added			
Ingredients			
Red Mark/Green Mark			

Labels	Any Other Product		
Name of the product			
Net Weight			
Price			
Date of manufacturing			
Date of expiry			
Product code			
Serving size			
Nutritive value per 100g Energy Protein Fat MUFA PUFA Trans Fat Sugar			
Preservative added			
Ingredients			
Red Mark/Green Mark			

EXERCISE 1

Q1. Define nutrition labelling

Q2. Write 5 advantages of nutrition label

Q3. Write the name of the companies which manufacture the organic Food

Q4. What is the difference between Pro Biotic and Pre Biotic?

Teacher's signature

PRACTICAL NO. 5

STANDARDISATION OF FOOD PRODUCTS

Aim: - To standardise food from each food group consumed in raw and cooked form

STANDARDISATION

Standardisation is a process by which a product is developed in such a manner that it produces same result on repeated production. Standardization is done to suit the requirement of the user and the use of standardized recipe is desirable to maintain the precise amount of nutrients and consistency in quantity and taste, texture and appearance.

It is a written formula for food preparation at anytime, anywhere.

SERVING SIZE

Serving size is the amount of food, which can be measured in terms of weigh, volume or number. Serving size is designed after assessing the portion sizes from food consumption survey to have a convenient measuring size with desired nutrient content.

One serving size is the amount of raw or cooked food set for each food exchange list or food group.

Serving size serve as a guide to understand and use the food pyramid, food exchange lists and nutritional facts on labels

Portion size is the amount of food a person chooses to eat at one sitting, whether it is a meal or a snack or beverage.

Unlike serving size, there is no standard portion size; it varies from person to person.

STANDARDISATION OF FOOD ITEMS

Food group/Food Item	Raw Measure	Cooked Measure	Medicinal Value	Side Effect on overconsumption
Milk & Milk Products				
Meat & Meat Product				

Food group/ Food Item	Raw Measure	Cooked Measure	Medicinal Value	Side Effect on overconsumption
Cereals				
Pulses				

Food group/Food Item	Raw Measure	Cooked Measure	Medicinal Value	Side Effect on overconsumption
Green leafy vegetables				
Roots and tubers				
Other vegetables				

Food group/Food Item	Raw Measure	Cooked Measure	Medicinal Value	Side Effect on overconsumption
Fruits				
Fats & Oils				
Sugars				

EXERCISE 1

Q1. Paste the pictures of measuring cup & spoon and write few lines about it

Q2. Mention the Standard measure of the following

1 teaspoon =

1 tablespoon =

1 cup =

1 glass =

1 katori =

Teacher's signature

PRACTICAL NO. 6

CALCULATION OF NUTRITIVE VALUE OF MILK & MILK PRODUCTS

Aim: - To plan, prepare and calculate the nutritive value of different products prepared using milk and milk products

1. Plan and prepare a Milk Based Porridge

    (a) Calculate the nutritive value of recipe

    (b) Write the difference between Full Cream Milk and Non-Dairy Milk

Meal	Menu	Ingredient	Amount	Energy	Protein	Fat

2. Plan and prepare a Kheer using Skim Milk
   (a) Calculate the nutritive value of recipe
   (b) Write the name of the test used to detect the purity of Milk

Meal	Menu	Ingredient	Amount	Energy	Protein	Fat

3. Plan and prepare dish using Paneer as an ingredient

   (a) Calculate the nutritive value of recipe

Meal	Menu	Ingredient	Amount	Energy	Protein	Fat

4. Plan and prepare a dish using Khoya

(a) Calculate the nutritive value of recipe

Meal	Menu	Ingredient	Amount	Energy	Protein	Fat

5. Plan and prepare a dish using Curd

   (a) Calculate the nutritive value of recipe

Meal	Menu	Ingredient	Amount	Energy	Protein	Fat

6. Plan and prepare a Pudding

(a) Calculate the nutritive value of recipe

Meal	**Menu**	**Ingredient**	**Amount**	**Energy**	**Protein**	**Fat**

7. Plan and prepare a Fruit Custard using Non- Dairy Milk
   (a) Calculate the nutritive value of recipe
   (b) Write the test used to test the presence of fat content in milk

Meal	Menu	Ingredient	Amount	Energy	Protein	Fat

Teachers Signature

PRACTICAL NO. 7

CALCULATION OF NUTRITIVE VALUE OF MEAT & MEAT PRODUCTS

Aim: - To plan, prepare and calculate the nutritive value of different food prepared using meat and meat products

1. Plan and prepare a scrambled Egg

   (a) Calculate the nutritive value of recipe

   (b) Write the nutritional benefits of egg

Meal	Menu	Ingredient	Amount	Energy	Protein	Fat

2. Plan and prepare a omelette

(a) Calculate the nutritive value of recipe

Meal	Menu	Ingredient	Amount	Energy	Protein	Fat

3. Plan and prepare a Poached Egg

   (a) Calculate the nutritive value of recipe

   (b) Write the nutritional benefits of poached egg

Meal	Menu	Ingredient	Amount	Energy	Protein	Fat

4. Plan a dish using fish as an ingredient

(a) Calculate the nutritive value of recipe

Meal	Menu	Ingredient	Amount	Energy	Protein	Fat

Teachers Signature

PRACTICAL NO. 8

CALCULATION OF NUTRITIVE VALUE OF CEREALS & PULSES

Aim:- To plan, prepare and calculate the nutritive value of different food products prepared using Cereals & Pulses

1. Plan and prepare a recipe using wheat

   (a) Calculate the nutritive value of recipe

   (b) Write the nutritive value of wheat

Meal	Menu	Ingredient	Amount	Energy	Protein	Fat

2. Plan and prepare a recipe using Rice

(a) Calculate the nutritive value of recipe

Meal	Menu	Ingredient	Amount	Energy	Protein	Fat

3. Plan and prepare a recipe using Maida
   (a) Calculate the nutritive value of recipe
   (b) Mention the name of 5 nutritious recipes that can be prepared using maida

Meal	**Menu**	**Ingredient**	**Amount**	**Energy**	**Protein**	**Fat**

4. Plan and prepare a recipe using Bread

   (a) Calculate the nutritive value of recipe

   (b) Write the difference between White Bread and Brown Bread

Meal	Menu	Ingredient	Amount	Energy	Protein	Fat

5. Plan and prepare a recipe using Oats
   (a) Calculate the nutritive value of recipe
   (b) Write the 5 benefits of oats and also mention the fibre content present in oats

Meal	**Menu**	**Ingredient**	**Amount**	**Energy**	**Protein**	**Fat**

6. Plan and prepare a recipe using Pulses

   (a) Calculate the nutritive value of recipe

   (b) Write the nutritional benefits of consuming pulses if a person do not eat Non- Veg

Meal	Menu	Ingredient	Amount	Energy	Protein	Fat

Teachers Signature

PRACTICAL NO. 9

CALCULATION OF NUTRITIVE VALUE OF VEGETABLES & FRUITS

Aim: - To plan, prepare and calculate the nutritive value of different products prepared using fruits and vegetables

1. Plan and prepare a recipe using Green Leafy Vegetables

   (a) Calculate the nutritive value of recipe

   (b) Write the advantages of consuming Green Leafy Vegetables

Meal	Menu	Ingredient	Amount	Energy	Protein	Fat

2. Plan and prepare a recipe made from Roots and Tubers

   (a) Calculate the nutritive value of recipe

   (b) Write the list of vegetables come under the category

Meal	Menu	Ingredient	Amount	Energy	Protein	Fat

3. Plan and prepare a recipe using Vegetables other than Green Leafy Vegetables and Roots & Tubers

   (a) Calculate the nutritive value of recipe

Meal	**Menu**	**Ingredient**	**Amount**	**Energy**	**Protein**	**Fat**

4. Plan and prepare a recipe using Fresh Fruits

   (a) Calculate the nutritive value of recipe

   (b) Write the nutritional benefits of consuming fresh fruits

Meal	**Menu**	**Ingredient**	**Amount**	**Energy**	**Protein**	**Fat**

5. Plan and prepare a recipe using Dry Stewed Fruits

   (a) Calculate the nutritive value of recipe

   (b) Write the name of Dry Stewed fruits available in market

Meal	**Menu**	**Ingredient**	**Amount**	**Energy**	**Protein**	**Fat**

6. Plan and prepare a Fruit Salad

   (a) Calculate the nutritive value of recipe

Meal	Menu	Ingredient	Amount	Energy	Protein	Fat

Teachers Signature

PRACTICAL NO. 10

CALCULATION OF NUTRITIVE VALUE OF BEVERAGES

Aim: - To plan, prepare and calculate the Nutritive Value of different Beverages

1. Plan and prepare a tea and coffee

   (a) Calculate the nutritive value of tea and coffee

   (b) Write the 5 side effects caused due to the overconsumption of tea and coffee

Meal	Menu	Ingredient	Amount	Energy	Protein	Fat

2. Plan and prepare a Fresh Fruit Juice for a Pregnant Mother
   (a) Calculate the nutritive value of fruit juice
   (b) Write the name of 5 Fruits that can be given in Pregnancy with their nutritional benefits

Meal	Menu	Ingredient	Amount	Energy	Protein	Fat

3. Plan and prepare 2 milk based beverage using toned milk and Non-Dairy Milk

   (a) Calculate the nutritive value of both the Beverages

   (b) Write the benefits of non-dairy milk

Meal	Menu	Ingredient	Amount	Energy	Protein	Fat

4. Plan and prepare a beverage containing Cocoa Powder
   (a) Calculate the nutritive value of the beverage
   (b) Write the name of the dishes in which cocoa powder is used

Meal	Menu	Ingredient	Amount	Energy	Protein	Fat

5. Plan and prepare a Milk Shake for a sports person

(a) Calculate the nutritive value of milk shake

Meal	Menu	Ingredient	Amount	Energy	Protein	Fat

Teachers Signature

PRACTICAL NO. 11

CALCULATION OF NUTRITIVE VALUE OF SOUPS

Aim: - To plan, prepare and calculate the nutritive value of different soups

1. Plan and prepare a Basic Soup

   (a) Calculate the nutritive value of recipe

Meal	Menu	Ingredient	Amount	Energy	Protein	Fat

2. Plan and prepare a Clear Soup
   (a) Calculate the nutritive value of recipe
   (b) Write in detail clear soups are given in which disease conditions

Meal	Menu	Ingredient	Amount	Energy	Protein	Fat

3. Plan and prepare a Cream Based Soup

   (a) Calculate the nutritive value of recipe

Meal	**Menu**	**Ingredient**	**Amount**	**Energy**	**Protein**	**Fat**

Teachers Signature

PRACTICAL NO. 12

CALCULATION OF NUTRITIVE VALUE OF SNACKS

Aim: - To plan, prepare and calculate the nutritive value of different snacks

1. Plan and prepare a dish using Rice Flakes

   (a) Calculate the nutritive value of recipe

Meal	Menu	Ingredient	Amount	Energy	Protein	Fat

2. Plan and prepare a Upma

   (a) Calculate the nutritive value of recipe

   (b) Write the nutritional value of semolina

Meal	**Menu**	**Ingredient**	**Amount**	**Energy**	**Protein**	**Fat**

3. Plan and prepare a Peanut Chikki

   (a) Calculate the nutritive value of recipe

Meal	Menu	Ingredient	Amount	Energy	Protein	Fat

4. Plan and prepare a Til Ladoo

   (a) Calculate the nutritive value of recipe

   (b) Write the nutritional values as well as benefits of Til

Meal	Menu	Ingredient	Amount	Energy	Protein	Fat

5. Plan and prepare a Cheese Toast

   (a) Calculate the nutritive value of recipe

Meal	Menu	Ingredient	Amount	Energy	Protein	Fat

6. Plan and prepare Pakoras using different ingredients
   (a) Calculate the nutritive value of recipe
   (b) Write the health hazards caused due to the over consumption of fried foods

Meal	**Menu**	**Ingredient**	**Amount**	**Energy**	**Protein**	**Fat**

Teachers Signature

Note: *Annexures and Bibliography of all 3 Parts are at the end of manual.*

PART - II

NUTRITION FOR LIFESPAN

DR. MONIKA ARORA

PRACTICAL NO. 1

INTRODUCTION TO FOOD EXCHANGE

Aim: - To learn and apply the knowledge of Food Exchange list in meal planning.

Food Exchange is a list of foods in a group with specified amount of food (weight/volume) having similar content of a given nutrient, i.e. similar amount of carbohydrate or fat or protein as the other foods included in the list. Food planners can select, mix and match foods from each exchange list as per food preferences cost and still have equivalent nutritional value.

Food Exchange helps to:

- Maintain the quantity of food, the total calories and provide a balanced diet.
- Provide the required amount of macronutrient and provide nutritious meal.
- Break the monotony in the meals, provide variety and flexibility in the diet and makes the diet interesting.

GENERAL DIETARY GUIDELINES

Right nutritional behaviour and dietary choices are needed to achieve dietary goals. The following dietary guidelines provide a broad framework for appropriate action:

- Eat variety of foods to ensure a balanced diet.

- Promote exclusive breastfeeding for six months and encourage breastfeeding till two years or as long as one can.
- Feed home-based semi solid foods to the infant after six months.
- Ensure adequate and appropriate diets for children and adolescents, both in health and sickness.
- Eat plenty of vegetables and fruits.
- Ensure moderate use of edible oils and animal foods.
- Avoid overeating to prevent overweight and obesity.
- Exercise regularly and be physically active to maintain ideal body weight.
- Ensure the use of safe and clean foods.
- Adopt right pre-cooking processes and appropriate cooking methods.
- Drink plenty of water and take carbonated beverages in moderation.
- Minimize the use of processed foods rich in salt, sugar and fats.
- Include micronutrient-rich foods in the diets of elderly people to enable them to be fit and active.

STEPS OF MEAL PLANNING

- Meal Planning starts with planning, considering a person's age, sex, gender and physiological conditions.
- The diet is generally divided into 3 major meals i.e. breakfast, lunch and dinner with a gap of 2-3 hours between each major meal 3-4 minor meals i.e. early morning, mid morning snacks, evening antioxidants rich tea should also be included in the diet to maintain the gap and fulfil the nutritional requirement of the individual.
- Small and frequent meals should be included. Once the personal data is collected, determine the RDA using ICMR table and calculated modified RDA as per the physiological status.

- Plan the menu by using food exchange provided in each meal for selecting specific foods.
- Draw a difference table with the standard.
- Interpretation

SAMPLE MENU- PLAN AND PREPARE A NORMAL DIET FOR A SEDENTARY WORKER

Step 1:- Record the personal data of the individual

- Name (optional)
- Age:- 25 years
- Gender:- male
- Height:- 5'6"
- Weight:- 60 kg
- Physical activity:- sedentary
- Physiological condition:- normal
- Food habits:- vegetarian
- Socio-economic status:- middle income group
- Food Allergy:- Egg (if any)

Step 2:- Determine the RDA by using ICMR

- Energy: - 2000 kcal Protein: - 60g
- Fats: - 25g

Step 3:- Estimate the amount of different Food Exchange

Food Group	Raw Amount		Exchange	Energy (kcal)	CHO (g)	Protein (g)	Fat (g)
Milk (skim)	320 ml	1 C	3	279	44.1	9	-
Pulse	30g	3Tbsp.	2	200	34	14	neg
Cereal/starch	20g	3Tbsp.	10.5	735	157.5	21	neg
Veg A	100	½ C	4	80	14	4	neg
Veg B	variable	-	3	120	21	6	neg
Fruit	variable	1 portion	3	135	30	neg	Neg
Fat	5g	1 tsp	6	270	-	-	30
Sugar	5g	1 tsp	4	80	20	-	-
Total				1900	321	60	30

Step 5:- Menu Planning

Meal	Menu	Ingredient	Amt	Exchange	Energy (kcal)	Protein (g)	CHO (g)	Fats (g)
Early Morning	Tea	Milk	½ cup	½	46.5	1.5	7.35	-
		Sugar	1 tsp	1	20	-	5	-
	Biscuit	Marie	2	2	140	4	30	-
Breakfast	2 Stuffed Parantha	Wheat flour	60g	2	140	4	30	-
		Cauliflower	20g	½	10	0.5	1.75	-
		Refined oil	2 tsp	2	90	-	-	10
Mid-Morning	Fruits	Banana	½	½	22.5	Neg	2.5	-
	Salad	Strawberry	1	1	45	Neg	5.0	-
		Grapes	½	½	22.5	Neg	2.5	-
		Apple	½	½	22.5	Neg	2.5	-
		Pomegranate	½	½	22.5	neg	2.5	-
Lunch	Salad	Cucumber	30g	½	10	0.5	1.75	-
	2 Chapatti	Multi grain atta	60g	2	140	4	30	-
		Arhar Dal	1 katori					
	Toor Dal	Onion	20g	1	100	7	17	-
		Tomato	30g	½	10	0.5	1.75	-
		Oil	1 tsp.	½	20	1	3.5	-
	Mix veg	Arbi	75g	1	45	-	-	5
		Corn	½ katori	1	40	2	7	-
				½	35	1	7.5	-
		Oil	1 tsp	1	45	-	-	5
	Curd	Plain curd	1katori	1	93	3	14.7	-
	White		½	1				

(Contd...)

Evening Tea	Tea	Milk	½ cup	½	46.5	1.5	7.35	-
		Sugar	1 tsp	1	20	-	5	-
	Sandwich	Brown Bread	2	2	140	4	30	-
		Onion	30g	½	10	0.5	1.75	-
		tomato	30g	½	20		3.5	-
Dinner	Macaroni	Macaroni	½ katori	½	35	1	7.5	-
	Salad	Tomato	20g	1	40	2	7	-
	Chapatti	Whole wheat atta	1	1	70	2	15	-
	Dal	Whole masoor dal	1 katori	1	100	7	17	-
		Oil	1tsp			-	-	5
		Capsicum		1	45			
		Potato	40g	1	40	2	7	-
	capsicum Veg	Oil	40g	1	20	2	7	-
			1tsp	1	45	-	-	5
Post Dinner	Milk	Double Toned milk	1 cup	1	93	3	14.7	-
		Sugar	1 tsp	1	20		5	-

EXERCISE 1

Plan a normal balanced diet for a female sedentary worker by using food exchange list.

Step 1:- Record the personal data of the individual

- Name
- Age:-
- Gender:-
- Height:-
- Weight:-
- Physical activity:-
- Physiological condition:-
- Food habits:-
- Socio-economic status:-

Step 2:- Determine the RDA by using ICMR

- Energy:-
- Protein:-
- Carbohydrate:-
- Fats:-

Step 3:- Estimate the amount of different Food Exchange

Food Group	Raw Amount		Exchange	Energy (kcal)	CHO (g)	Protein (g)	Fat (g)
	gram/ ml	Household measures					
Total							

Step 4:-Detailed Menu Plan

Meal	Menu	Ingredient	Amount	Exchange	Energy (kcal)	Protein (g)	CHO (g)	Fats (g)

Meal	Menu	Ingredient	Amt	Exchange	Energy (kcal)	Protein (g)	CHO (g)	Fats (g)

Meal	Menu	Ingredient	Amt	Exchange	Energy (kcal)	Protein (g)	CHO (g)	Fats (g)

Difference Table-

Nutrients	Standard RDA	Modified RDA	Calculated Plan	Difference(±)
Energy				
Proteins				
Carbohydrates				
Fats				

Interpretation

....

....

....

....

....

....

....

....

Dietary Guidelines

-

-

-

-

Teachers Signature

PRACTICAL NO. 2

PLANNING OF NORMAL DIET

Aim: - To plan and prepare a normal balanced diet for a sedentary worker

STEP 1:- PERSONAL INFORMATION

- Name:-
- Age:-
- Height:-
- Weight:-
- BMI:-
- Type of Worker
- Physiological Condition:-
- Socio-Economic Status:-
- Food Allergy:-

STEP 2:- RDA FROM ICMR

- Energy:-
- Protein:-
- CHO:-
- Fats:-

Step 3:- Estimate the amount of different Food Exchange

Food Group	Raw Amount		Exchange	Energy (kcal)	CHO (g)	Protein (g)	Fat (g)
	gram/ ml	Household measures					
Total							

Step 4:- Detailed Menu Plan

Meal	Menu	Ingredient	Amount	Exchange	Energy (kcal)	Protein (g)	CHO (g)	Fats (g)

Meal	Menu	Ingredient	Amount	Exchange	Energy (kcal)	Protein (g)	CHO (g)	Fats (g)

Meal	Menu	Ingredient	Amount	Exchange	Energy (kcal)	Protein (g)	CHO (g)	Fats (g)

TOTAL-

Step 5:- Difference Table

Nutrients	Standard RDA	Modified RDA	Calculated Plan	Difference(±)
Energy				
Proteins				
Carbohydrates				
Fats				

Interpretation

....
....
....
....
....
....
....
....

Dietary Guidelines

-

-

-

-

Teachers Signature

EXERCISE 1

Q1. Mention the activities that come under the following categories

Sedentary worker	Moderate worker	Heavy worker

Q2. Define Balance Diet

....

....

....

....

Q3. Write the name of the low cost nutritious food items that can be given in normal diet

....

....

Teachers Signature

PRACTICAL NO. 3

BALANCE DIET FOR PREGNANT WOMEN

Aim:- To plan and prepare a normal balanced diet for a Pregnant Woman.

Foetal growth and pregnancy demand additional nutrients, and these requirements are defined in the new dietary reference intakes (DRIs), which include adequate intakes (AIs) and RDA's.

ENERGY

Additional energy is required during pregnancy to support the metabolic demands of pregnancy and foetal growth. Metabolism increases by 15% in pregnancy. The 2002 DRIs for energy for the pregnant female are the same as for the non pregnant female in the first trimester but then increase an additional 340 to 350 kcal/day during the second trimester and another 112 kcal/day in the third trimester.

PROTEIN

There is an additional protein requirement for a pregnant woman to support the synthesis of maternal and foetal tissues, but the magnitude of this increase is uncertain. Protein requirement increases throughout gestation and is maximum during the third trimester. The current RDA of 0.66 g/kg/day of protein for pregnant women are the same as that for the non pregnant women in the first half of pregnancy and increases for the second half to 71 g/day. For each additional foetus another 25 g/day of protein is recommended.

CARBOHYDRATES

For the first time, DRIs for carbohydrates in pregnancy is represented. The estimated average requirement (EAR) is 135 g/day, and the AI is 175 g/day. This 135 to 175g /day is the recommended amount to provide enough calories in the diet to prevent ketosis and maintain appropriate blood glucose during pregnancy.

FIBRE

Daily consumption of whole-grain breads and cereals, leafy green and yellow vegetables, and fresh and dried fruits should be encouraged to provide additional minerals, vitamins, and fibre. The DRI for fibre during pregnancy is 28 g/day.

LIPIDS

There is no DRI for lipids during pregnancy. The amount of fat in the diet should depend on energy requirements for proper weight gain.

FOLIC ACID

Folic acid requirements increase during pregnancy in response to the demands of maternal erythropoiesis and foetal and placental growth and, most important, for the prevention of NTDs. The RDA for folic acid in pregnancy is 600 mcg, a 200 mcg increase over that for non pregnant females. The IOM (Institute of Medicine) recommends that 400 mcg of the 600 mcg/day be provided by folate-fortified foods or supplements as it is better absorbed.

Step 1:- Personal Information

- Name:-
- Age:-
- Height:-
- Weight:-
- BMI:-
- Type of Worker
- Socio-Economic Status:-
- Food Allergy:-

Step 2:- RDA from ICMR

- Energy:-
- Protein:-
- CHO:-
- Fats:-

Step 3:- Estimate the amount of different Food Exchange

Food Group	**Raw Amount**		**Exchange**	**Energy (kcal)**	**CHO (g)**	**Protein (g)**	**Fat (g)**
	gram/ ml	**Household measures**					
Total							

Step 4:-Detailed Menu Plan

Meal	Menu	Ingredient	Amount	Exchange	Energy (kcal)	Protein (g)	CHO (g)	Fats (g)

Meal	Menu	Ingredient	Amount	Exchange	Energy (kcal)	Protein (g)	CHO (g)	Fats (g)

Step: 5. Difference Table

Nutrients	Standard RDA	Modified RDA	Calculated Plan	Difference(±)
Energy				
Proteins				
Carbohydrates				
Fats				

Interpretation

....

....

....

....

....

....

....

Dietary Guidelines

-

-

-

Teachers Signature

EXERCISE-2

Q1. Write the name of nutrients and their sources which are important during pregnancy.

....

....

....

....

....

....

....

....

Q2. Mention the food myths which are avoided and given in pregnancy. Justify by giving proper explanation.

....

....

....

....

....

....

....

....

....

Teachers Signature

PRACTICAL NO. 4

DIET IN PREGNANCY

Aim: - To plan and prepare a normal balanced diet for a expected woman suffering from Gestational Diabetes.

Step 1:- Personal Information

- Name:-
- Age:-
- Height:-
- Weight:-
- BMI:-
- Type of Worker
- Physiological Condition:-
- Socio-Economic Status:-
- Food Allergy:-

Step 2:- RDA from ICMR

- Energy:-
- Protein:-
- CHO:-
- Fats:-

Step 3:- Estimate the amount of different Food Exchange

Food Group	Raw Amount		Exchange	Energy (kcal)	CHO (g)	Protein (g)	Fat (g)
	gram/ ml	Household measures					
Total							

Step 4:-Detailed Menu Plan

Meal	Menu	Ingredient	Amount	Exchange	Energy (kcal)	Protein (g)	CHO (g)	Fats (g)

Meal	Menu	Ingredient	Amount	Exchange	Energy (kcal)	Protein (g)	CHO (g)	Fats (g)

Meal	Menu	Ingredient	Amount	Exchange	Energy (kcal)	Protein (g)	CHO (g)	Fats (g)

TOTAL

Step 5:- Diffference Table

Nutrients	**Standard RDA**	**Modified RDA**	**Calculated Plan**	**Difference(±)**
Energy				
Proteins				
Carbohydrates				
Fats				

Interpretation

....

....

....

....

....

....

....

....

....

Dietary Guidelines

-
-
-
-

Teachers Signature

PRACTICAL NO. 5

DIET FOR LACTATING WOMEN

Aim: - To plan and prepare a normal balanced diet for a Lactating Mother.

Step 1:- Personal Information

- Name:-
- Age:-
- Height:-
- Weight:-
- BMI:-
- Type of Worker
- Physiological Condition:-
- Socio-Economic Status:-
- Food Allergy:-

Step 2:- RDA from ICMR

- Energy:-
- Protein:-
- CHO:-
- Fats:-

Step 3:- Estimate the amount of different Food Exchange

Food Group	Raw Amount		Exchange	Energy (kcal)	CHO (g)	Protein (g)	Fat (g)
	gram/ ml	Household measures					
Total							

Step 4:- Detailed Menu Plan

Meal	Menu	Ingredient	Amount	Exchange	Energy (kcal)	Protein (g)	CHO (g)	Fats (g)

Meal	Menu	Ingredient	Amount	Exchange	Energy (kcal)	Protein (g)	CHO (g)	Fats (g)

Meal	Menu	Ingredient	Amount	Exchange	Energy (kcal)	Protein (g)	CHO (g)	Fats (g)

TOTAL-

Step: 5. Difference Table

Nutrients	Standard RDA	Modified RDA	Calculated Plan	Difference(±)
Energy				
Proteins				
Carbohydrates				
Fats				

Interpretation

....

....

....

....

....

....

....

Dietary Guidelines

-

-

-

-

Teachers Signature

EXERCISE-3

Q1. Write the name of the nutrients with their requirement which are important for lactating women.

....

....

....

....

....

....

....

....

....

....

Q2. Write the advantages of exclusive breast feeding.

....

....

....

....

....

....

....

....

....

Teachers Signature

PRACTICAL NO. 6

WEANING DIET

Aim: - Plan and prepare a weaning balanced chart for an Infant (0-6months).

Nutrient needs of infants reflect rates of growth, energy expended in activity, basal metabolic needs, and the interaction of the nutrients consumed

Energy

Full-term infants who are breast-fed to satiety and infants who are fed a standard 21 kcal/ oz formula generally adjust their intake to meet their energy needs. The recently developed World Health Organization (WHO) Growth Standards use the breastfed infant as the normative model for "prescriptive" assessment of infant growth.

Protein

Protein is needed for tissue replacement, deposition of lean body mass, and growth. Protein requirements during the rapid growth of infancy are higher per kilogram of weight than those for adults or older children. Recommendation for protein intake is based on the composition of human milk, and it is assumed that the efficiency of human milk use is 100%.

Lipids

The current recommendation for infants younger than one year of age is to consume a minimum of 30 g of fat/day. This quantity is present in human milk and all infant formulas.

Carbohydrates

Carbohydrates should supply 30% to 60% of the energy intake during infancy. Approximately 40% of the energy in human milk and 40% to 50% of the energy in infant formulas is derived from lactose or other carbohydrates.

Step 1:- Personal Information

- Name:-
- Age:-
- Height:-
- Weight:-
- BMI:-
- Type of Worker-
- Physiological Condition:-
- Socio-Economic Status:-
- Food Allergy:-

Step 2:- RDA from ICMR

- Energy:-
- Protein:-
- CHO:-
- Fats:-

Step 3:-Feeding Pattern/Frequency

Breast milk	Quantity (ml)	Bottle milk	Quantity (ml)

Interpretation

....

....

....

....

....

....

....

....

....

....

Dietary Guidelines

-
-
-
-

EXERCISE-4

Q1. Define Weaning Food and its importance.

....

....

....

....

....

....

Teachers Signature

PRACTICAL NO. 7

WEANING DIET

Aim: - Plan and prepare a weaning balanced chart for an Infant (6-12months).

Step 1:- Personal Information

- Name:-
- Age:-
- Height:-
- Weight:-
- BMI:-
- Type of Worker-
- Physiological Condition:-
- Socio-Economic Status:-
- Food Allergy:-

Step 2:- RDA from ICMR

- Energy:-
- Protein:-
- CHO:-
- Fats:-

Step 3:- Estimate the amount of different Food Exchange

Food Group	Raw Amount		Exchange	Energy (kcal)	CHO (g)	Protein (g)	Fat (g)
	gram/ ml	Household measures					
Total							

Step 4:-Detailed Menu Plan

Meal	Menu	Ingredient	Amount	Exchange	Energy (kcal)	Protein (g)	CHO (g)	Fats (g)

Meal	Menu	Ingredient	Amount	Exchange	Energy (kcal)	Protein (g)	CHO (g)	Fats (g)

Meal	Menu	Ingredient	Amount	Exchange	Energy (kcal)	Protein (g)	CHO (g)	Fats (g)

TOTAL-

Step:5. Difference Table

Nutrients	Standard RDA	Modified RDA	Calculated Plan	Difference(±)
Energy				
Proteins				
Carbohydrates				
Fats				

Interpretation

....

....

....

....

....

....

....

Dietary Guidelines

-
-
-
-

Teachers Signature

EXERCISE - 5

Q1. Write the foods that can be given as complementary food.

....

....

....

....

....

....

....

....

....

....

Q2. Write the direction for home preparation of infant food.

....

....

....

....

....

....

....

....

....

....

Teachers Signature

PRACTICAL NO. 8

DIET FOR PRE-SCHOOL CHILDREN

Aim: - To plan and prepare a balance diet for a Pre-School Going Children (——years old).

Step 1:- Personal Information

- Name:-
- Age:-
- Height:-
- Weight:-
- BMI:-
- Type of Worker-
- Physiological Condition:-
- Socio-Economic Status:-
- Food Allergy:-

Step 2:- RDA from ICMR

- Energy:-
- Protein:-
- CHO:-
- Fats:-

Step 3:- Estimate the amount of different Food Exchange

Food Group	Raw Amount		Exchange	Energy (kcal)	CHO (g)	Protein (g)	Fat (g)
	gram/ ml	Household measures					
Total							

Step 4:- Detailed Menu Plan

Meal	Menu	Ingredient	Amount	Exchange	Energy (kcal)	Protein (g)	CHO (g)	Fats (g)

Meal	Menu	Ingredient	Amount	Exchange	Energy (kcal)	Protein (g)	CHO (g)	Fats (g)

Meal	Menu	Ingredient	Amount	Exchange	Energy (kcal)	Protein (g)	CHO (g)	Fats (g)

Step 5. Difference Table

Nutrients	Standard RDA	Modified RDA	Calculated Plan	Difference(±)
Energy				
Proteins				
Carbohydrates				
Fats				

Interpretation

....

....

....

....

....

....

....

....

Dietary Guidelines

-
-
-
-

Teachers Signature

PRACTICAL NO. 9

DIET FOR SCHOOL CHILD

Aim: - To plan and prepare a balance diet for a School Child (.....years old).

Step 1:- Personal Information

- Name:-
- Age:-
- Height:-
- Weight:-
- BMI:-
- Type of Worker-
- Physiological Condition:-
- Socio-Economic Status:-
- Food Allergy:-

Step 2:- RDA from ICMR

- Energy:-
- Protein:-
- CHO:-

Step 3:- Estimate the amount of different Food Exchange

Food Group	Raw Amount		Exchange	Energy (kcal)	CHO (g)	Protein (g)	Fat (g)
	gram/ ml	Household measures					
Total							

Step 4:-Detailed Menu Plan

Meal	Menu	Ingredient	Amount	Exchange	Energy (kcal)	Protein (g)	CHO (g)	Fats (g)

Meal	Menu	Ingredient	Amount	Exchange	Energy (kcal)	Protein (g)	CHO (g)	Fats (g)

Meal	Menu	Ingredient	Amount	Exchange	Energy (kcal)	Protein (g)	CHO (g)	Fats (g)

TOTAL-

Step: 5. Difference Table

Nutrients	Standard RDA	Modified RDA	Calculated Plan	Difference(±)
Energy				
Proteins				
Carbohydrates				
Fats				

Interpretation

....

....

....

....

....

....

....

....

....

Dietary Guidelines

-
-
-
-

EXERCISE - 9

Q. PLAN AND PREPARE A NUTRITIOUS PACKED LUNCH FOR A SCHOOL CHILD AND ALSO CALCULATE ITS ENERGY AND PROTEIN CONTENT.

....

....

....

....

....

....

....

....

....

....

....

....

....

....

....

....

....

....

....

....

—Teachers Signature

PRACTICAL NO. 10

DIET FOR ADOLESCENCE

Aim: - To plan and prepare a Nutritious Balance Diet for Adolescence.

Step 1:- Personal Information

- Name:-
- Age:-
- Height:-
- Weight:-
- BMI:-
- Type of Worker-
- Physiological Condition:-
- Socio-Economic Status:-
- Food Allergy:-

Step 2:- RDA from ICMR

- Energy:-
- Protein:-
- CHO:-
- Fats:-

Step 3:- Estimate the amount of different Food Exchange

Food Group	Raw Amount		Exchange	Energy (kcal)	CHO (g)	Protein (g)	Fat (g)
	gram/ ml	Household measures					
Total							

Step 4:- Detailed Menu Plan

Meal	Menu	Ingredient	Amount	Exchange	Energy (kcal)	Protein (g)	CHO (g)	Fats (g)

Meal	Menu	Ingredient	Amount	Exchange	Energy (kcal)	Protein (g)	CHO (g)	Fats (g)

Meal	Menu	Ingredient	Amount	Exchange	Energy (kcal)	Protein (g)	CHO (g)	Fats (g)

TOTAL-

Step: 5. Difference Table

Nutrients	Standard RDA	Modified RDA	Calculated Plan	Difference(±)
Energy				
Proteins				
Carbohydrates				
Fats				

Interpretation

....

....

....

....

....

....

....

Dietary Guidelines

-
-
-
-

Teachers Signature

EXERCISE-7

Q1. Write the feeding problems which are faced by an adolescent

....

....

....

....

....

....

....

....

....

....

Q1. Define the term Eating Disorders

....

....

....

....

....

....

....

....

....

Teachers Signature

PRACTICAL NO. 11

DIET FOR ADULT

Aim: - To plan and prepare a balance diet for an Adult belonging to different Income Group

1. **Plan and prepare a nutritious Balance Diet for a male who is a heavy worker and belongs to Lower Income Group.**

Step 1:- Personal Information

- Name:-
- Age:-
- Height:-
- Weight:-
- BMI:-
- Type of Worker-
- Physiological Condition:-
- Socio-Economic Status:-
- Food Allergy:-

Step 2:- RDA from ICMR

- Energy:-
- Protein:-
- CHO:-
- Fats:-

Step 3:- Estimate the amount of different Food Exchange

Food Group	Raw Amount		Exchange	Energy (kcal)	CHO (g)	Protein (g)	Fat (g)
	gram/ ml	Household measures					
Total							

Step 4:- Detailed Menu Plan

Meal	Menu	Ingredient	Amount	Exchange	Energy (kcal)	Protein (g)	CHO (g)	Fats (g)

Meal	Menu	Ingredient	Amount	Exchange	Energy (kcal)	Protein (g)	CHO (g)	Fats (g)

Meal	Menu	Ingredient	Amount	Exchange	Energy (kcal)	Protein (g)	CHO (g)	Fats (g)

TOTAL-

Step: 5. Difference Table

Nutrients	Standard RDA	Modified RDA	Calculated Plan	Difference(±)
Energy				
Proteins				
Carbohydrates				
Fats				

Interpretation

....

....

....

....

....

....

....

....

....

Dietary Guidelines

-
-
-
-

Teachers Signature

Q2. Plan and prepare a nutritious Balance Diet for a female who is a moderate worker and belongs to Middle Income Group

Step 1:- Personal Information

- Name:-
- Age:-
- Height:-
- Weight:-
- BMI:-
- Type of Worker-
- Physiological Condition:-
- Socio-Economic Status:-
- Food Allergy:-

Step 2:- RDA from ICMR

- Energy:-
- Protein:-
- CHO:-
- Fats:-

Step 3:- Estimate the amount of different Food Exchange

Food Group	Raw Amount		Exchange	Energy (kcal)	CHO (g)	Protein (g)	Fat (g)
	gram/ ml	Household measures					
Total							

Step 4:- Detailed Menu Plan

Meal	Menu	Ingredient	Amount	Exchange	Energy (kcal)	Protein (g)	CHO (g)	Fats (g)

Meal	Menu	Ingredient	Amount	Exchange	Energy (kcal)	Protein (g)	CHO (g)	Fats (g)

Meal	Menu	Ingredient	Amount	Exchange	Energy (kcal)	Protein (g)	CHO (g)	Fats (g)

TOTAL-

Step: 5. Difference Table

Nutrients	Standard RDA	Modified RDA	Calculated Plan	Difference(±)
Energy				
Proteins				
Carbohydrates				
Fats				

Interpretation

....

....

....

....

....

....

....

....

....

Dietary Guidelines

-

-

Teachers Signature

PRACTICAL NO. 12

DIET FOR SENIOR CITIZEN

Aim: - To plan and prepare a Nutritious Balance Diet for a Senior Citizen belonging to .... Income Group.

Step 1:- Personal Information

- Name:-
- Age:-
- Height:-
- Weight:-
- BMI:-
- Type of Worker-
- Physiological Condition:-
- Socio-Economic Status:-
- Food Allergy:-

Step 2:- RDA from ICMR

- Energy:-
- Protein:-
- CHO:-
- Fats:-

Step 3:- Estimate the amount of different Food Exchange

Food Group	Raw Amount		Exchange	Energy (kcal)	CHO (g)	Protein (g)	Fat (g)
	gram/ ml	Household measures					
Total							

Step 4:- Detailed Menu Plan

Meal	Menu	Ingredient	Amount	Exchange	Energy (kcal)	Protein (g)	CHO (g)	Fats (g)

Meal	Menu	Ingredient	Amount	Exchange	Energy (kcal)	Protein (g)	CHO (g)	Fats (g)

Meal	Menu	Ingredient	Amount	Exchange	Energy (kcal)	Protein (g)	CHO (g)	Fats (g)

TOTAL-

Step: 5. Difference Table

Nutrients	Standard RDA	Modified RDA	Calculated Plan	Difference(±)
Energy				
Proteins				
Carbohydrates				
Fats				

Interpretation

....

....

....

....

....

....

....

....

....

Dietary Guidelines

-
-

Teachers Signature

Note: *Annexures and Bibliography of all 3 Parts are at the end of manual.*

PART - III

THERAPEUTIC NUTRITION

MS. SWAYAM SIDDHA

PRACTICAL NO. 1

STANDARDIZATION OF COMMON FOOD PREPARATIONS

Aim:- To standardize and prepare the food preparations form different food groups

STANDARDIZATION

Standardization is a process by which a product is developed in such a manner that it produces same result on repeated production. Standardization is done to suit the requirement of the user and the use of standardized recipe is desirable to maintain the precise amount of nutrients and consistency in quantity and taste, texture and appearance.

It is a written formula for food preparation at anytime, anywhere.

Q1. To standardize and prepare a dish using milk & milk product for a school children who is on normal diet

1. **To standardize and prepare a dish using milk**

   Name of Recipe: - **Category:-**

   Serving Size: - **Preparation Time:-**

   Cooking Time:-

S.no	Ingredient	Amount	Energy (Kcal)	Protein (g)	Fats (g)	CHO (g)
Total						

Method:-

2. To standardize and prepare a dish using milk product

Name of Recipe: - **Category:-**

Serving Size: - **Preparation Time:-**

Cooking Time:-

S.no	Ingredient	Amount	Energy (Kcal)	Protein (g)	Fats (g)	CHO (g)
Total						

Method:-

Q2. To standardize and prepare a dish using egg for a fracture patient

Name of Recipe: - **Category:-**

Serving Size: - **Preparation Time:-**

Cooking Time:-

S.no	Ingredient	Amount	Energy (Kcal)	Protein (g)	Fats (g)	CHO (g)
Total						

Method:-

Q3. To standardize and prepare a dish using Cereals and Pulses

Name of Recipe: - **Category:-**

Serving Size: - **Preparation Time:-**

Cooking Time:-

S.no	Ingredient	Amount	Energy (Kcal)	Protein (g)	Fats (g)	CHO (g)
	Total					

Method:-

Q4. To standardize and prepare a dish using vegetables for a Diabetic patient

Name of Recipe: - **Category:-**

Serving Size: - **Preparation Time:-**

Cooking Time:-

S.no	**Ingredient**	**Amount**	**Energy (Kcal)**	**Protein (g)**	**Fats (g)**	**CHO (g)**
Total						

Method:-

Q5. To standardize and prepare a dish using high fibre fruits for an obese patient

Name of Recipe:- **Category:-**

Serving Size:- **Preparation Time:-**

Cooking Time:-

S.no	**Ingredient**	**Amount**	**Energy (Kcal)**	**Protein (g)**	**Fats (g)**	**CHO (g)**
Total						

Method:-

EXERCISE: - 1

Q1. Write the difference between Portion Size and Serving Size

Q2. Write the importance of standardization

Q3. What are the points that need to kept in mind to prevent nutrition loss while cooking

Teachers Signature

PRACTICAL NO. 2

PLANNING OF NORMAL DIET

Aim:- To plan and prepare a normal diet for a 45 year male moderate worker,vegetarian,Ht:- 157cm and wt:- 60 kg and belongs to middle income group

Personal Information:-

- Age:-
- Ht:-
- Wt:-
- BMI:-
- Physical activity:-
- Food Habits:-
- Physiological condition:-
- Socio-Economic Status:-

Estimation of RDA

- Energy:-
- Protein:-
- Fat:-

Calculation of Food Exchange

Food Group	Raw Amount		Exchange	Energy (Kcal)	CHO (g)	Protein (g)	Fat (g)
Milk (skim)							
Pulse							
Cereal/starch							
Veg A							
Veg B							
Fruit							
Fat							
Sugar							
Total							

Distribution of Exchange

Food Group	No of Exchange	Early Morning	Break fast	Mid-Morning	Lunch	Evening tea	Dinner	Post-Dinner
Milk (skim)								
Pulse								
Cereal/ starch								
Veg A								
Veg B								
Fruit								
Fat								
Sugar								

Menu Plan

Meal	Menu	Ingredient	Amt	Exchange	Energy (Kcal)	Protein (g)	CHO (g)	Fats (g)

Meal	Menu	Ingredient	Amt	Exchange	Energy (Kcal)	Protein (g)	CHO (g)	Fats (g)

EXERCISE: - 1

Q1. Write the factors to be considered while planning normal diet

Q2. Write the nutritional consideration of normal diet

Teachers Signature

PRACTICAL NO. 3

PLANNING OF CLEAR LIQUID AND LIQUID DIET

Aim:- To plan and prepare a clear liquid diet & liquid diet for a sedentary worker

1. Plan and prepare a clear liquid diet for a patient suffering from typhoid

Personal Information

- Age:-
- Physical activity:-
- Food Habits:-
- Physiological condition:-
- Socio-Economic Status:-

Estimation of RDA

- Energy:-
- Protein:-
- Fat:-

Menu Plan

Meal	Menu	Ingredient	Amt	Energy (Kcal)	Protein (g)	CHO (g)	Fats (g)
6 am							
8 am							
10 am							
12 noon							
2 pm							
4 pm							
6 pm							
8 pm							
10 pm							

EXERCISE 1

Q1. Write the foods that are given and avoided in clear liquid diet

Q2. Write the nutritional factors of clear liquid diet

Q3. Write the food sources that are beneficial for the patient. Mention the nutrients and their nutritive value as well

2. Plan and prepare a liquid diet for a patient suffering from water & electrolyte imbalance

Personal Information

- Age:-
- Physical activity:-
- Food Habits:-
- Physiological condition:-
- Socio-Economic Status:-

Estimation of RDA

- Energy:-
- Protein:-
- Fat:-
- Other important nutrient:-

Menu Plan

Meal	Menu	Ingredient	Amt	Energy (Kcal)	Protein (g)	CHO (g)	Fats (g)
6am							
8am							
10 am							
12 noon							
2 pm							
4 pm							
6 pm							
8 pm							
10 pm							

EXERCISE 2

Q1. Write the foods that are given and avoided in liquid diet

Q2. Write the difference between clear and liquid diet

Q3. Write the food sources that can be given to these kinds of patients. Mention the nutrients present and their nutritive value.

Teachers Signature

PRACTICAL NO. 4

PLANNING OF SOFT DIET

Aim:- To plan and prepare a soft diet for a 18 year female patient suffering from diarrhoea. The pateint is a non-vegetarian,Ht:- 160cm and wt:- 56 kg and belongs to lower income group

Personal Information:-

- Age:-
- Ht:-
- Wt:-
- BMI:-
- Physical activity:-
- Food Habits:-
- Physiological condition:-
- Socio-Economic Status:-

Estimation of RDA	**Modified RDA**
• Energy:-	Energy:-
• Protein:-	Protein:-
• Fat:-	Fat:-

Calculation of Food Exchange

Food Group	Raw Amount		Exchange	Energy (Kcal)	CHO (g)	Protein (g)	Fat (g)
Milk (skim)							
Meat							
Pulse							
Cereal/starch							
Veg A							
Veg B							
Fruit							
Fat							
Sugar							
Total							

Distribution of Exchange

Food Group	No of Exchange	Early Morning	Break fast	Mid-Morning	Lunch	Evening tea	Dinner	Post-Dinner
Milk								
Meat								
Pulse								
Cereal								
Veg A								
Veg B								
Fruit								
Fat								
Sugar								

Menu Plan

Meal	Menu	Ingredient	Amt	Exchange	Energy (Kcal)	Protein (g)	CHO (g)	Fats (g)

Meal	**Menu**	**Ingredient**	**Amt**	**Exchange**	**Energy (Kcal)**	**Protein (g)**	**CHO (g)**	**Fats (g)**

EXERCISE: - 1

Q1 Plan a semi-solid diet for a patient who underwent a dental surgery

Teachers Signature

PRACTICAL NO. 5

PLANNING OF TUBE FEED

Aim:- To plan and prepare tube feed for the patient

1. Plan and prepare a 100 ml * 2 hourly tube feed for a patient suffering from CVA

Personal Information

- Ht:-
- Wt:-
- BMI:-
- Physiological condition:-
- Socio-Economic Status:-

Estimation of RDA

- Energy:-
- Protein:-
- Fat:-

Menu Plan

Meal	Menu	Energy (Kcal)	Protein (g)	CHO (g)	Fats (g)
6am					
8am					
10 am					
12 noon					
2 pm					
4 pm					
6 pm					
8 pm					
10 pm					

2. Plan and prepare a 150 ml * 2 hourly tube feed for a patient suffering from diabetes and meningitis

Personal Information

- Ht:-
- Wt:-
- BMI:-
- Physiological condition:-
- Socio-Economic Status:-

Estimation of RDA

- Energy:-
- Protein:-
- Fat:-

Menu Plan

Meal	Menu	Energy (Kcal)	Protein (g)	CHO (g)	Fats (g)
6am					
8am					
10 am					
12 noon					
2 pm					
4 pm					
6 pm					
8 pm					
10 pm					

3. Plan and prepare a 200 ml * 2 hourly high protein tube feed for an unconscious road accident patient

Personal Information

- Ht:-
- Wt:-
- BMI:-
- Physiological condition:-
- Socio-Economic Status:-

Estimation of RDA

- Energy:-
- Protein:-
- Fat:-
- CHO:-

Menu Plan

Meal	Menu	Energy (Kcal)	Protein (g)	CHO (g)	Fats (g)
6am					
8am					
10 am					
12 noon					
2 pm					
4 pm					
6 pm					
8 pm					
10 pm					

4. Plan and prepare a 250 ml * 2 hourly tube feed for a patient suffering from Chronic Renal Faliure

Personal Information

- Ht:-
- Wt:-
- BMI:-
- Physiological condition:-
- Socio-Economic Status:-

Estimation of RDA

- Energy:-
- Protein:-
- Fat:-

Menu Plan

Meal	Menu	Energy (Kcal)	Protein (g)	CHO (g)	Fats (g)
6am					
8am					
10 am					
12 noon					
2 pm					
4 pm					
6 pm					
8 pm					
10 pm					

5. Plan and prepare a 300 ml * 3 hourly tube feed for a patient suffering from Chronic Renal Faliure

Personal Information

- Ht:-
- Wt:-
- BMI:-
- Physiological condition:-
- Socio-Economic Status:-

Estimation of RDA

- Energy:-
- Protein:-
- Fat:-

Meal	Menu	Energy (Kcal)	Protein (g)	CHO (g)	Fats (g)
6am					
9am					
12 noon					
3 pm					
6 pm					
9 pm					

EXERCISE 1

Q1. Write the points that need to be considered while planning and serving tube feed

Q2. Write the name of different tube feeds which can be given to a patient.

Teachers Signature

PRACTICAL NO. 6

PLANNING OF DIET

Aim:- To plan and prepare a high calorie normal diet for a underweight school boy,vegetarian and belongs to lower income group

Personal Information:-

- Age:-
- Ht:-
- Wt:-
- BMI:-
- Physical activity:-
- Food Habits:-
- Physiological condition:-
- Socio-Economic Status:-

Estimation of RDA

- Energy:-
- Protein:-
- Fat:-

Modified RDA

Energy:-

Protein:-

Fat:-

Calculation of Food Exchange

Food Group	Raw Amount		Exchange	Energy (Kcal)	CHO (g)	Protein (g)	Fat (g)
Milk (skim)							
Pulse							
Cereal/starch							
Veg A							
Veg B							
Fruit							
Fat							
Sugar							
Total							

Distribution of Exchange

Food Group	No of Exchange	Early Morning	Break fast	Mid-Morning	Lunch	Evening tea	Dinner	Post-Dinner
Milk (skim)								
Pulse								
Cereal/ starch								
Veg A								
Veg B								
Fruit								
Fat								
Sugar								

Menu Plan

Meal	Menu	Ingredient	Amt	Exchange	Energy (Kcal)	Protein (g)	CHO (g)	Fats (g)

Meal	Menu	Ingredient	Amt	Exchange	Energy (Kcal)	Protein (g)	CHO (g)	Fats (g)

EXERCISE: - 1

Q1. Write the factors to be considered while planning high calorie diet

Q2. Write the food sources which are high in calorie. Mention their nutritive value as well

Q3. List the name of diseases which are more common in an underweight patient

1. To plan and prepare a low calorie normal diet for a 60 year old female obese patient who is a sedentary worker,non-vegetarian,Ht:- 155cm and wt:- 95kg and belongs to higher income group

Personal Information:-

- Age:-
- Ht:-
- Wt:-
- BMI:-
- Physical activity:-
- Food Habits:-
- Physiological condition:-
- Socio-Economic Status:-

Estimation of RDA	**Modified RDA**
• Energy:-	Energy:-
• Protein:-	Protein:-
• Fat:-	Fat:-

Calculation of Food Exchange

Food Group	**Raw Amount**		**Exchange**	**Energy (Kcal)**	**CHO (g)**	**Protein (g)**	**Fat (g)**
Milk (skim)							
Pulse							
Cereal/starch							
Veg A							
Veg B							
Fruit							
Fat							
Sugar							
Total							

Distribution of Exchange

Food Group	**No of Exchange**	**Early Morning**	**Break fast**	**Mid-Morning**	**Lunch**	**Evening tea**	**Dinner**	**Post-Dinner**
Milk (skim)								
Pulse								
Cereal/ starch								
Veg A								
Veg B								
Fruit								
Fat								
Sugar								

Menu Plan

Meal	Menu	Ingredient	Amt	Exchange	Energy (Kcal)	Protein (g)	CHO (g)	Fats (g)

Meal	**Menu**	**Ingredient**	**Amt**	**Exchange**	**Energy (Kcal)**	**Protein (g)**	**CHO (g)**	**Fats (g)**

EXERCISE:- 2

Q1. Write the factors to be considered while planning low calorie diet

Q2. Write the food sources which are high in calorie. Mention their nutritive value as well

Q3. Write the health hazards of obesity

Teachers Signature

PRACTICAL NO. 7

PLANNING OF BLAND DIET

Aim:- To plan and prepare a bland soft diet for a 25 year old female patient suffering from peptic ulcer.

Personal Information:-

- Age:-
- Ht:-
- Wt:-
- BMI:-
- Physical activity:-
- Food Habits:-
- Physiological condition:-
- Socio-Economic Status:-

Estimation of RDA	**Modified RDA**
• Energy:-	Energy:-
• Protein:-	Protein:-
• Fat:-	Fat:-

Calculation of Food Exchange

Food Group	Raw Amount		Exchange	Energy (Kcal)	CHO (g)	Protein (g)	Fat (g)
Milk (skim)							
Pulse							
Cereal/starch							
Veg A							
Veg B							
Fruit							
Fat							
Sugar							
Total							

Distribution of Exchange

Food Group	No of Exchange	Early Morning	Break fast	Mid-Morning	Lunch	Evening tea	Dinner	Post-Dinner
Milk (skim)								
Pulse								
Cereal/ starch								
Veg A								
Veg B								
Fruit								
Fat								
Sugar								

Menu Plan

Meal	Menu	Ingredient	Amt	Exchange	Energy (Kcal)	Protein (g)	CHO (g)	Fats (g)

Meal	Menu	Ingredient	Amt	Exchange	Energy (Kcal)	Protein (g)	CHO (g)	Fats (g)

EXERCISE: - 1

Q1. Define Bland diet

Q2. Write the foods avoided in Bland diet

Q3. Draw and write the foods that are avoided and given (in moderate & good amount) to a Peptic Ulcer patient

Teachers Signature

PRACTICAL NO. 8

DIET FOR VIRAL HEPATITIS

Aim:- To plan and prepare a normal diet for a 62 year old male patient suffering from viral hepatitis.

Personal Information:-

- Age:-
- Ht:-
- Wt:-
- BMI:-
- Physical activity:-
- Food Habits:-
- Physiological condition:-
- Socio-Economic Status:-

Estimation of RDA	**Modified RDA**
• Energy:-	Energy:-
• Protein:-	Protein:-
• Fat:-	Fat:-

Calculation of Food Exchange

Food Group	Raw Amount		Exchange	Energy (Kcal)	CHO (g)	Protein (g)	Fat (g)
Milk (skim)							
Pulse							
Cereal/starch							
Veg A							
Veg B							
Fruit							
Fat							
Sugar							
Total							

Distribution of Exchange

Food Group	No of Exchange	Early Morning	Break fast	Mid-Morning	Lunch	Evening tea	Dinner	Post-Dinner
Milk (skim)								
Pulse								
Cereal/ starch								
Veg A								
Veg B								
Fruit								
Fat								
Sugar								

Menu Plan

Meal	Menu	Ingredient	Amt	Exchange	Energy (Kcal)	Protein (g)	CHO (g)	Fats (g)

Meal	Menu	Ingredient	Amt	Exchange	Energy (Kcal)	Protein (g)	CHO (g)	Fats (g)

EXERCISE: - 1

Q1. What is the relationship between viral hepatitis and Iron?

Q2. Write the foods avoided in hepatitis

Q3. Why sugar and salt intake is limited in this condition?

Teachers Signature

PRACTICAL NO. 9

DIET FOR DIABETES

Aim:- To plan and prepare a normal diet for a 15 year old boy patient suffering from Type I Diabetes Mellitus.

Personal Information:-

- Age:-
- Ht:-
- Wt:-
- BMI:-
- Physical activity:-
- Food Habits:-
- Physiological condition:-
- Socio-Economic Status:-

Estimation of RDA	**Modified RDA**
• Energy:-	Energy:-
• Protein:-	Protein:-
• Fat:-	Fat:-

Calculation of Food Exchange

Food Group	Raw Amount		Exchange	Energy (Kcal)	CHO (g)	Protein (g)	Fat (g)
Milk (skim)							
Meat							
Pulse							
Cereal/starch							
Veg A							
Veg B							
Fruit							
Fat							
Total							

Distribution of Exchange

Food Group	No of Exchange	Early Morning	Break fast	Mid-Morning	Lunch	Evening tea	Dinner	Post-Dinner
Milk (skim)								
Meat								
Pulse								
Cereal/ starch								
Veg A								
Veg B								
Fruit								
Fat								

Menu Plan

Meal	Menu	Ingredient	Amt	Exchange	Energy (Kcal)	Protein (g)	CHO (g)	Fats (g)

Meal	**Menu**	**Ingredient**	**Amt**	**Exchange**	**Energy (Kcal)**	**Protein (g)**	**CHO (g)**	**Fats (g)**

EXERCISE: - 1

Q1. Define Type I diabetes mellitus

Q2. Write the foods avoided in type 1 diabetes

1. To plan and prepare a normal diet for a 30 year old pregnant women suffering from Gestational Diabetes Mellitus.

Personal Information:-

- Age:-
- Ht:-
- Wt:-
- BMI:-
- Physical activity:-
- Food Habits:-
- Physiological condition:-
- Socio-Economic Status:-

Estimation of RDA	Modified RDA
• Energy:-	Energy:-
• Protein:-	Protein:-
• Fat:-	Fat:-

Calculation of Food Exchange

Food Group	Raw Amount		Exchange	Energy (Kcal)	CHO (g)	Protein (g)	Fat (g)
Milk (skim)							
Meat							
Pulse							
Cereal/starch							
Veg A							
Veg B							
Fruit							
Fat							
Total							

Distribution of Exchange

Food Group	No of Exchange	Early Morning	Break fast	Mid-Morning	Lunch	Evening tea	Dinner	Post-Dinner
Milk (skim)								
Meat								
Pulse								
Cereal/ starch								
Veg A								
Veg B								
Fruit								
Fat								

Menu Plan

Meal	Menu	Ingredient	Amt	Exchange	Energy (Kcal)	Protein (g)	CHO (g)	Fats (g)

Meal	Menu	Ingredient	Amt	Exchange	Energy (Kcal)	Protein (g)	CHO (g)	Fats (g)

EXERCISE: - 2

Q1. Define Gestational diabetes mellitus

Q2. Write the normal sugar level for pregnant women

2. To plan and prepare a normal diet for a 70 year old sedentary male worker suffering from Type II Diabetes Mellitus.

Personal Information:-

- Age:-
- Ht:-
- Wt:-
- BMI:-
- Physical activity:-
- Food Habits:-
- Physiological condition:-
- Socio-Economic Status:-

Estimation of RDA	Modified RDA
• Energy:-	Energy:-
• Protein:-	Protein:-
• Fat:-	Fat:-

Calculation of Food Exchange

Food Group	Raw Amount		Exchange	Energy (Kcal)	CHO (g)	Protein (g)	Fat (g)
Milk (skim)							
Meat							
Pulse							
Cereal/starch							
Veg A							
Veg B							
Fruit							
Fat							
Total							

Distribution of Exchange

Food Group	No of Exchange	Early Morning	Break fast	Mid-Morning	Lunch	Evening tea	Dinner	Post-Dinner
Milk (skim)								
Meat								
Pulse								
Cereal/ starch								
Veg A								
Veg B								
Fruit								
Fat								

Menu Plan

Meal	Menu	Ingredient	Amt	Exchange	Energy (Kcal)	Protein (g)	CHO (g)	Fats (g)

Meal	Menu	Ingredient	Amt	Exchange	Energy (Kcal)	Protein (g)	CHO (g)	Fats (g)

EXERCISE:- 3

Q1. Write the relationship of fibre and diabetes

Q2. Write the difference between glycemic load and glycemic index

Teachers Signature

PRACTICAL NO. 10

DIET FOR CARDIOVASCULAR DISEASE

Aim:- To plan and prepare a low fat normal diet for a 80 year old male sedentary patient, Ht:- 5'6", Wt:- 55kg, Eggatarian suffering from hypertension and atherosclerosis.

Personal Information:-

- Age:-
- Ht:-
- Wt:-
- BMI:-
- Physical activity:-
- Food Habits:-
- Physiological condition:-
- Socio-Economic Status:-

Estimation of RDA	**Modified RDA**
• Energy:-	Energy:-
• Protein:-	Protein:-
• Fat:-	Fat:-

Calculation of Food Exchange

Food Group	**Raw Amount**		**Exchange**	**Energy (Kcal)**	**CHO (g)**	**Protein (g)**	**Fat (g)**
Milk (skim)							
Pulse							
Cereal/starch							
Veg A							
Veg B							
Fruit							
Fat							
Sugar							
Total							

Distribution of Exchange

Food Group	**No of Exchange**	**Early Morning**	**Break fast**	**Mid-Morning**	**Lunch**	**Evening tea**	**Dinner**	**Post-Dinner**
Milk (skim)								
Pulse								
Cereal/ starch								
Veg A								
Veg B								
Fruit								
Fat								
Sugar								

Menu Plan

Meal	Menu	Ingredient	Amt	Exchange	Energy (Kcal)	Protein (g)	CHO (g)	Fats (g)

Meal	Menu	Ingredient	Amt	Exchange	Energy (Kcal)	Protein (g)	CHO (g)	Fats (g)

EXERCISE: - 1

Q1. Write the difference between saturated and unsaturated fats

Q2. Write the risk factors of cardiovascular disease

Q3. Write the food sources that help in lowering the cholesterol level

Q4. Write the foods that are avoided for a hypertensive patient

Teachers Signature

PRACTICAL NO. 11

DIET FOR RENAL DISEASE

Aim:- To plan and prepare a low protein soft diet for a heavy worker, Ht:- 5'9", Wt:- 70kg, non-vegetarian suffering from Chronic Renal Failure .

Personal Information:-

- Age:-
- Ht:-
- Wt:-
- BMI:-
- Physical activity:-
- Food Habits:-
- Physiological condition:-
- Socio-Economic Status:-

Estimation of RDA	Modified RDA
• Energy:-	Energy:-
• Protein:-	Protein:-
• Fat:-	Fat:-

Calculation of Food Exchange

Food Group	Raw Amount		Exchange	Energy (Kcal)	CHO (g)	Protein (g)	Fat (g)
Milk (skim)							
Pulse							
Cereal/starch							
Veg A							
Veg B							
Fruit							
Fat							
Sugar							
Total							

Distribution of Exchange

Food Group	No of Exchange	Early Morning	Break fast	Mid-Morning	Lunch	Evening tea	Dinner	Post-Dinner
Milk (skim)								
Pulse								
Cereal/ starch								
Veg A								
Veg B								
Fruit								
Fat								
Sugar								

Menu Plan

Meal	Menu	Ingredient	Amt	Exchange	Energy (Kcal)	Protein (g)	CHO (g)	Fats (g)

Meal	Menu	Ingredient	Amt	Exchange	Energy (Kcal)	Protein (g)	CHO (g)	Fats (g)

EXERCISE: - 1

Q1. Write the ways by which potassium can be leached out form the foods and then used for a renal disease patient

Q2. Write the factors to be considered while planning and cooking diet for such patient

Q3. Write the difference between acute renal failure and chronic renal failure

1. To plan and prepare a high protein normal diet for a patient with Ht:- 5'4", Wt:- 50kg, vegetarian suffering from Nephrotic Syndrome.

Personal Information:-

- Age:-
- Ht:-
- Wt:-
- BMI:-
- Physical activity:-
- Food Habits:-
- Physiological condition:-
- Socio-Economic Status:-

Estimation of RDA	**Modified RDA**
• Energy:-	Energy:-
• Protein:-	Protein:-
• Fat:-	Fat:-

Calculation of Food Exchange

Food Group	Raw Amount		Exchange	Energy (Kcal)	CHO (g)	Protein (g)	Fat (g)
Milk (skim)							
Pulse							
Cereal/starch							
Veg A							
Veg B							
Fruit							
Fat							
Sugar							
Total							

Distribution of Exchange

Food Group	No of Exchange	Early Morning	Break fast	Mid-Morning	Lunch	Evening tea	Dinner	Post-Dinner
Milk (skim)								
Pulse								
Cereal/ starch								
Veg A								
Veg B								
Fruit								
Fat								
Sugar								

Menu Plan

Meal	Menu	Ingredient	Amt	Exchange	Energy (Kcal)	Protein (g)	CHO (g)	Fats (g)

Meal	Menu	Ingredient	Amt	Exchange	Energy (Kcal)	Protein (g)	CHO (g)	Fats (g)

EXERCISE: - 2

Q1. Define Nephrotic Syndrome

Q2. Write the foods given and avoided in nephritic syndrome

Q3. Discuss the relationship of sodium and potassium with nephrotic syndrome

Q4. Write the normal renal parameters and the renal parameters of a patient suffering from renal disease

2. To plan and prepare a liquid diet for a patient with Ht:- 5'5", Wt:- 60kg, vegetarian suffering from Acute Renal Failure and his oral intake is very minimum.

Personal Information:-

- Age:-
- Ht:-
- Wt:-
- BMI:-
- Physical activity:-
- Food Habits:-
- Physiological condition:-
- Socio-Economic Status:-

Estimation of RDA	**Modified RDA**
• Energy:-	Energy:-
• Protein:-	Protein:-
• Fat:-	Fat:-

Menu Plan

Meal	Menu	Ingredient	Amt	Energy (Kcal)	Protein (g)	CHO (g)	Fats (g)
6am							
8am							
10 am							
12 noon							
2 pm							
4 pm							
6 pm							
8 pm							
10 pm							

EXERCISE: - 3

Q1. Write the foods that are rich in sodium & potassium that should be avoided for a renal patient

Q2. Write food sources that are rich in nutrients other than the nutrients restricted in renal disease and can be given to such patients to fulfil their nutritional requirement

Teachers Signature

PRACTICAL NO. 12

PLANNING OF LOW COST NUTRITIOUS DIET

Aim:- To plan and prepare a low cost high protein snack for a child suffering from PEM

Personal Information:-

- Age:-
- Food Habits:-
- Physiological condition:-
- Socio-Economic Status:-

Estimation of RDA	**Modified RDA**
• Energy:-	Energy:-
• Protein:-	Protein:-
• Fat:-	Fat:-

Menu Plan

Meal	Menu	Ingredient	Amt	Exchange	Energy (Kcal)	Protein (g)	CHO (g)	Fats (g)

EXERCISE: - 1

Q1. Define PEM. Write the nutritional requirement of a child suffering from PEM

Q2. Write the factors to be considered while planning and cooking diet for such patient

1. To plan and prepare a medium cost snack for a 30 year old lactating women suffering from Anemia

Personal Information:-

- Age:-
- Food Habits:-
- Physiological condition:-
- Socio-Economic Status:-

Estimation of RDA	**Modified RDA**
• Energy:-	Energy:-
• Protein:-	Protein:-
• Fat:-	Fat:-

Menu Plan

Meal	Menu	Ingredient	Amt	Exchange	Energy (Kcal)	Protein (g)	CHO (g)	Fats (g)

EXERCISE: - 2

Q1. Define Anaemia

Q2. Write the factors to be considered while cooking to prevent the iron loss

Q3. Write the foods which are good and best sources of iron

2. To plan and prepare a snack for a patient suffering from Vitamin A Deficiency

Personal Information:-

- Age:-
- Food Habits:-
- Physiological condition:-
- Socio-Economic Status:-

Estimation of RDA	**Modified RDA**
• Energy:-	Energy:-
• Protein:-	Protein:
• Fat:-	Fat:-
	Vitamin A:-

Menu Plan

Meal	Menu	Ingredient	Amt	Exchange	Energy (Kcal)	Protein (g)	CHO (g)	Fats (g)

EXERCISE: - 3

Q1. Write the foods which are good and best sources of Vitamin A

Q2. Write the normal nutritional requirement of Vitamin A as well for a person suffering from its deficiency disease.

Teachers Signature

PRACTICAL NO. 13

DIET FOR CELIAC SPRUE

Aim:- To plan and prepare a diet for a male moderate worker suffering from gluten enteropathy/ celiac sprue

Personal Information:-

- Age:-
- Ht:-
- Wt:-
- BMI:-
- Physical activity:-
- Food Habits:-
- Physiological condition:-
- Socio-Economic Status:-

Estimation of RDA	**Modified RDA**
• Energy:-	Energy:-
• Protein:-	Protein:-
• Fat:-	Fat:-

Calculation of Food Exchange

Food Group	Raw Amount		Exchange	Energy (Kcal)	CHO (g)	Protein (g)	Fat (g)
Milk (skim)							
Pulse							
Cereal/starch							
Veg A							
Veg B							
Fruit							
Fat							
Sugar							
Total							

Distribution of Exchange

Food Group	No of Exchange	Early Morning	Break fast	Mid-Morning	Lunch	Evening tea	Dinner	Post-Dinner
Milk (skim)								
Pulse								
Cereal/ starch								
Veg A								
Veg B								
Fruit								
Fat								
Sugar								

Menu Plan

Meal	Menu	Ingredient	Amt	Exchange	Energy (Kcal)	Protein (g)	CHO (g)	Fats (g)

Meal	Menu	Ingredient	Amt	Exchange	Energy (Kcal)	Protein (g)	CHO (g)	Fats (g)

EXERCISE: - 1

Q1. Define Celiac Disease

Q2. Write the biochemical test used to detect celiac disease

Q3. Write the foods that are totally avoided for such kind of patients

Q4. Write the foods that can be given to fulfil the nutritional requirement of the patient

EXERCISE:- 2

Q1. Plan and prepare a low cost nutritious snack for a celiac disease patient. Calculate the cost of the snack

Menu Plan

Meal	Menu	Ingredient	Amt	Exchange	Energy (Kcal)	Protein (g)	CHO (g)	Fats (g)

Calculation of cost of snack

Interpretation

....
....
....
....
....

Teachers Signature

Note: *Annexures and Bibliography of all 3 Parts are at the end of manual.*

ANNEXURES

ANNEXURE-I
RDA FOR INDIANS BY ICMR

Group	Particulars	Body Wt. (kg)	Net Energy (kcal/d)	Protein (g/d)	Visible fat (g/d)	Calcium (mg/d)	Iron (mg/d)	Vitamin A (µg/d)		Thiamine (mg/d)	Riboflavin (mg/d)	Niacin – equivalent (mg/d)	Pyridoxine (mg/d)	Ascorbic acid (mg/d)	Dietary folate (µg/d)	Vit. B12 (µg/d)	Magn- esium (mg /d)	Zinc (mg /d)
								Retinol	β Carotene									
Man	sedentary work	60	2320	60	25	600	17	600	4800	1.2	1.4	16	2	40	200	1	340	12
	moderate work		2730		30					1.4	1.6	18						
	heavy work		3490		40					1.7	2.1	21						
Woman	sedentary work	55	1900	55	20	600	21	600	4800	1	1.1	12	2	40	200	1	310	10
	moderate work		2230		25					1.1	1.3	14						
	heavy work		2850		30					1.4	1.7	16						
	pregnant women		350	82.2	30	1200	35	800	6400	0.2	0.3	2	2.5	60	500	1.2		12
	lactation 0-6m		600	77.9	30	1200	25	950	7600	0.3	0.4	4	2.5	50	300	1.5		
	lactation 6-12 m		520	70.2	30					0.2	0.3	3	2.5					
Infants	0-6 months	5.4	92 kcal /kg /d	1.16 g /kg /d		500	46 µg /kg /d	350	2800	0.2	0.3	710 µg /kg	0.1	25	25	0.2	30	
	6-12 months	8.4	80 kcal /kg /d	1.69 g/ kg /d	19		5			0.3	0.4	650 µg /kg	0.4				45	
Children	1-3 years	12.9	1060	16.7	27	600	9	400	3200	0.5	0.6	8	0.9	40	80	0.2-1.0	50	5
	4-6 years	18	1350	20.1	25		13			0.7	0.8	11	0.9		100		70	7
	7-9 years	25.1	1690	29.5	30		16	600	4800	0.8	1	13	1.6		120		100	8
Boys	10-12 years	34.3	2190	39.9	35	800	21	600	4800	1.1	1.3	15	1.6	40	140	0.2-1.0	120	9
Girls	10-12 years	35	2010	40.4	35		27			1	1.2	13	1.6				160	9
Boys	13-15 years	47.6	2750	54.3	45		32			1.4	1.6	16	2	40	150	0.2-1.0	165	11
Girls	13-15 years	46.6	2330	51.9	40		27			1.2	1.4	14	2				210	11
Boys	16-17 years	55.4	3020	61.5	50		28			1.5	1.8	17	2	40	200	0.2-1.0	195	12
Girls	16-17 years	52.1	2440	55.5	35		26			1	1.2	14	2				235	1

ANNEXURES II

Reference Body Weights of Indians Employed for Computing RDA, 2009

Group	Age	Reference Body Weight (kg)
Adult man	18-29 y	60.0
Adult woman (NPNL)	18-29 y	55.0
Infants	0-6 m	5.4*
	6 – 12 m	8.4*
Children	1 – 3 y	12.9*
	4 – 6 y	18.0
	7 – 9 y	25.1
Boys	10 - 12 y	34.3
	13 – 15 y	47.6
	16 – 17 y	55.4
Girls	10 - 12 y	35.0
	13 – 15 y	46.6
	16 – 17 y	52.1

ANNEXURE-III
Protein, fat and energy deposition during growth in the first year of life

Age (months)	Protein gain g/d	Fat mass gain g/d	Weight gain g/d	Energy accrued in normal growth*	
				KJ/g	kcal/g
Boys					
0-3	2.6	19.6	32.7	25.1	6.0
3-6	2.3	3.9	17.7	11.6	2.8
6-9	2.3	0.5	11.8	6.2	1.5
9-12	1.6	1.7	9.1	11.4	2.7
Girls					
0-3	2.2	19.7	31.1	26.2	6.3
3-6	1.9	5.8	17.3	15.6	3.7
6-9	2.0	0.8	17.3	7.4	1.8
9-12	1.8	1.1	8.7	9.8	2.3

* Energy equivalents of 1 g protein = 23.6 KJ (5.65 kcal); 1 g fat = 38.7 KJ (9.25 kcal)

ANNEXURES IV

Energy Requirement of Indian Men and Women at Different Ages and Body Weights

Sex	Body Weight Kg	Age 18-30 yrs				Age 30-60 yrs				Age > 60 years		
		BMR kcal	Sedentary Work kcal	Moderate Work kcal	Heavy Work kcal	BMR kcal	Sedentary Work kcal	Moderate Work kcal	Heavy Work kcal	BMR kcal	Sedentary Work kcal	Moderate Work kcal
MALES	45	1298	1986	2336	2985	1324	2026	2383	3045	1039	1590	1870
	50	1370	2096	2466	3151	1358	2078	2444	3123	1103	1688	1985
	55	1443	2208	2597	3319	1433	2196	2579	3296	1167	1786	2101
	60	1515	2318	2727	3485	1487	2275	2671	3420	1231	1883	2216
	65	1588	2430	2858	3652	1542	2359	2736	3547	1295	1981	2331
	70	1660	2540	2988	3818	1596	2442	2873	3671	1359	2079	2446
	75	1773	2716	3191	4078	1651	2526	2971	3797	1423	2177	2565
FEMALES	40	1031	1577	1856	2371	1120	1714	2016	2576	965	1477	1737
	45	1101	1685	1982	2532	1162	1778	2092	2673	1015	1553	1627
	50	1171	1792	2108	2693	1203	1841	2165	2767	1065	1630	1917
	55	1241	1899	2234	2854	1245	1905	2241	2864	1115	1706	2007
	60	1311	2006	2360	3015	1286	1966	2315	2958	1165	1782	2097
	65	1381	2113	2486	3176	1328	2032	2390	3054	1215	1860	2187
	70	1451	2220	2612	3337	1369	2095	2464	3149	1265	1936	2277

ANNEXURES V
Balanced Diet for Adults - Sedentary/ Moderate/ Heavy Activity (Number of portions)

Type of Worker							
	g/portion	Sedentary		Moderate		Heavy	
		Man	Woman	Man	Woman	Man	Woman
		No. of portions					
Cereals & millets	30	12.5	9	15	11	20	16
Pulses	30	2.5	2	3	2.5	4	3
Milk & milk products	100 ml	3	3	3	3	3	3
Roots & Tubers	100	2	2	2	2	2	2
Green leafy vegetables	100	1	1	1	1	1	1
Other Vegetables	100	2	2	2	2	2	2
Fruits	100	1	1	1	1	1	1
Sugar	**5**	4	4	6	6	11	9
Fat	**5**	5	4	6	5	8	6

To calculate the day's requirement of above mentioned food groups for an individual, multiply grams per portion with number of portions

ANNEXURES VI

Balanced Diet for Infants, Children and Adolescents (Number of Portions)

Food Groups	g/portion	Infant 6-12 months	1-3	4-6	7-9	Years					
						10-12		13-15		16-18	
						Girls	Boys	Girls	Boys	Girls	Boys
Cereals & millets	30	0.5	2	4	6	8	10	11	14	11	15
Pulses	30	0.25	1	1.0	2	2	2	2	2.5	2.5	3
Milk & milk products	100 ml	4[a]	5	5	5	5	5	5	5	5	5
Roots & Tubers	100	0.5	0.5	1	1	1	1	1	1.5	2	2
Green leafy vegetables	100	0.25	0.5	0.5	1	1	1	1	1	1	1
Other Vegetables	100	0.25	0.5	1	1	2	2	2	2	2	2
Fruits	100	1	1	1	1	1	1	1	1	1	1
Sugar	5	2	3	4	4	6	6	5	4	5	6
Fat	5	4	5	5	6	7	7	8	9	7	10

[a] Quantity indicates top milk. For breastfed infants, 200 ml top milk is required.
One portion of pulse may be exchanged with one portion (50 g) of egg/meat/chicken/fish.
For infants introduce egg/meat/chicken/fish around 9 months.

ANNEXURES VII
Food Pyramid

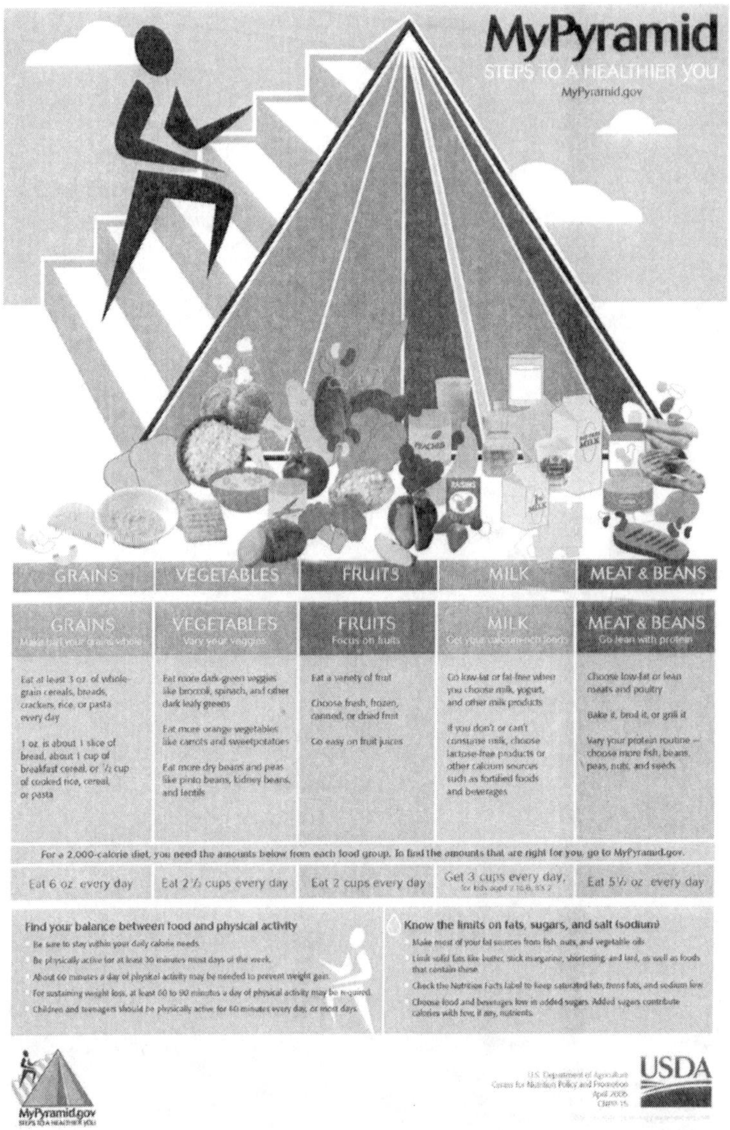
MyPyramid
STEPS TO A HEALTHIER YOU
MyPyramid.gov
GRAINS
VEGETABLES
FRUITS
MILK
MEAT & BEANS
GRAINS
VEGETABLES
Vary your veggies
FRUITS
Focus on fruits
MILK
MEAT & BEANS
Go lean with protein
Eat at least 3 oz. of whole-grain cereals, breads, crackers, rice, or pasta every day
1 oz. is about 1 slice of bread, about 1 cup of breakfast cereal, or ½ cup of cooked rice, cereal, or pasta
Eat more dark-green veggies like broccoli, spinach, and other dark leafy greens
Eat more orange vegetables like carrots and sweetpotatoes
Eat more dry beans and peas like pinto beans, kidney beans, and lentils
Eat a variety of fruit
Choose fresh, frozen, canned, or dried fruit
Go easy on fruit juices
Go low-fat or fat-free when you choose milk, yogurt, and other milk products
If you don't or can't consume milk, choose lactose-free products or other calcium sources such as fortified foods and beverages
Choose low-fat or lean meats and poultry
Bake it, broil it, or grill it
Vary your protein routine — choose more fish, beans, peas, nuts, and seeds
For a 2,000-calorie diet, you need the amounts below from each food group. To find the amounts that are right for you, go to MyPyramid.gov.
Eat 6 oz. every day
Eat 2½ cups every day
Eat 2 cups every day
Get 3 cups every day;
Eat 5½ oz. every day
Find your balance between food and physical activity
Be sure to stay within your daily calorie needs.
Be physically active for at least 30 minutes most days of the week.
About 60 minutes a day of physical activity may be needed to prevent weight gain.
For sustaining weight loss, at least 60 to 90 minutes a day of physical activity may be required.
Children and teenagers should be physically active for 60 minutes every day, or most days.
Know the limits on fats, sugars, and salt (sodium)
Make most of your fat sources from fish, nuts, and vegetable oils.
Limit solid fats like butter, stick margarine, shortening, and lard, as well as foods that contain these.
Check the Nutrition Facts label to keep saturated fats, trans fats, and sodium low.
Choose food and beverages low in added sugars. Added sugars contribute calories with few, if any, nutrients.
MyPyramid.gov
U.S. Department of Agriculture
Center for Nutrition Policy and Promotion
April 2005
USDA

ANNEXURES VIII
Approximate Calorific Value of Nuts, Salads and Fruits

	Portions	Calories
	Nuts	
Almonds	10 Nos.	85
Cashew nuts	10 Nos.	95
Coconut (fresh)	100 g	444
Coconut (dry)	100 g	662
Peanuts	50 Nos.	90
	Fresh fruits	
Apple	1 medium	65
Banana	1 medium	90
Grapes	30 Nos.	70
Guava	1 medium	50
Jackfruit	4 pieces	90
Mango	1 medium	180
Mosambi/orange	1 medium	40
Papaya	1 pieces	80
Pineapple	1 pieces	50
Sapota	1 medium	80
Custard apple	1 medium	130
Watermelon/muskmelon	1 slice	15
	Salads	

(Contd...)

Beetroot	1 medium	30
Carrot	1 medium	70
Cucumber	1 medium	12
Onion	1 medium	25
Radish	1 medium	10
Tomato	1 medium	10

ANNEXURES IX
Low Calorie Vegetables and Fruits (20 Kcal)

Name of the vegetable	Calories/ 100gm
Green Leafy Vegetables	
Amaranth (stem)	19
Ambat chukka	15
Celery stalk	18
Spinach stalk	20
Roots & Tubers	
Radish table	16
Radish white	17
Other vegetables	
Ash gourd	10
Bottle gourd	12
Cluster beans	16
Colocasia stem	18
Cucumber	13
Ghosala	18
Kovai	18
Parwal	20
Ridge guard	17
Snake guard	18
Vegetable marrow	17

(Contd...)

Fruits	
Bilimbi	19
Jamb safed	19
Musk melon	17
Water melon	16
Orange juice	9
Tomato ripe	20

ANNEXURES X
Vegetables and Fruits with High Calorie Value (> 100Kcal)

Name of the vegetable	Calories/ 100gm
Green Leafy Vegetables	
Chekkur manis	103
Colocasia leaves (dried)	277
Curry leaves	108
Fetid cassia (dried) (Chakunda)	292
Rape leaves (dried)	297
Tamarind leaves	115
Roots & Tubers	
Arrow root flour	334
Parsnip	101
Sweet potato	120
Tapioca	157
Yam ordinary	111
Yam wild	110
Other vegetables	
Beans, scarlet runner	158
Jack fruit, seeds	133
Karonda (dry)	364
Lotus stem (dry)	234
Sundakai (dry)	269

(*Contd...*)

Water chestnut (fresh)	115
Water chestnut (dry)	330
Fruits	
Apricot (dry)	306
Avacado pear	215
Banana	116
Bael fruit	116
Currants, red	316
Dates (dried)	317
Dates fresh	144
Mahua (ripe)	111
Raisins	308
Seetaphal	104
Wood apple	134

ANNEXURES XI
Approximate Calorific Value of Some Cooked Preparations

Preparation	Quantity for one serving	Calories (Kcal)
1. Cereal		
Rice	1 cup	170
Phulka	1 No.	80
Paratha	1 No.	150
Puri	1 No.	80
Bread	2 slices	170
Poha	1 cup	270
Upma	1 cup	270
Idli	2 Nos.	150
Dosa	1 No.	125
Kichidi	1 cup	200
Wheat porridge	1 cup	220
Semolina porridge	1 cup	220
Cereal flakes with milk (corn/wheat/rice)	1 cup	220
2. Pulse		
Plain dhal	½ cup	100
Sambar	1 cup	110
3. Vegetable		

(*Contd...*)

With gravy	1 cup	170
Dry	1 cup	150
4. Non-Vegetarian		
Boiled egg	1 No	90
Ommelette	1 No	160
Fried egg	1 No	160
Mutton curry	¾ cup	260
Chicken curry	¾ cup	240
Fish fried	2 big pieces	190
Fish cutlet	2 Nos.	190
Prawn curry	¾ cup	220
Keema kofta curry	¾ cup(6 small koftas)	240
5. Savoury snacks		
Bajji or pakora	8 Nos.	280
Besan ka pura	1 No.	220
Chat (Dahi-pakori)	5 pieces	220
Cheese balls	2 Nos.	250
Dahi vada	2 Nos.	180
Vada	2 Nos.	140
Masala vada	2 Nos.	150
Masala dosa	1 No.	200
Pea-kachori	2 Nos.	380
Potato bonda	2 Nos.	200

(*Contd...*)

Sago vada	2 Nos.	210
Samosa	1 No.	200
Sandwiches (butter - 2tbsp)	2 Nos.	200
Vegetable puff	1 No.	200
Pizza (Cheese and tomato)	1 slice	200
6. Chutneys		
Coconut/groundnuts/til	2 tbsp	120
Tomato	1 tbsp	10
Tamarind (w it h jaggery)	1 tbsp	60
7. Sweets and Desserts		
Besan barfi	2 small pieces	400
Chikki	2 pieces	290
Fruit cake	1 pieces	270
Rice puttu	½ cup	280
Sandesh	2 Nos.	140
Double ka meetha	½ cup	280
Halwa (kesari)	½ cup	320
Jelly/Jam	1 tbsp	20
Custard (caramel)	½ cup	160
Srikhand	½ cup	380
Milk chocolate	25 g	140

(*Contd...*)

Ice-cream	½ cup	200
8. Beverages		
Tea (2 tsp sugar +50 ml toned milk)	1 cup	75
Coffee (2 tsp sugar + 100 ml)	1 cup	110
Cow's milk (2 tsp sugar)	1 cup	180
Buffalo's milk (2 tsp sugar)	1 cup	320
Lassi (2 tsp sugar)	1 cup/glass (200 ml)	110
Squash	1 cup/glass	75
Syrups (Sharabats)	1 cup/glass	200
Cold drinks	1 bottle (200 ml)	150
Fresh lime juice	1 glass	60

ANNEXURES XII
Glycemic Index (GI) of Common Foods

s.no	Name of the foods	Glycemic Index	s.no	Name of the foods	Glycemic Index
1	White wheat bread	75 + 2	17	Mango (raw)	51 + 5
2	Whole wheat bread	74 + 2	18	Watermelon (raw)	76 + 4
3	Wheat roti	62 + 3	19	Potato (boiled)	78 + 4
4	Chapatti	52 +4	20	French fries (potato)	63 + 5
5	White boiled rice	73 + 4	21	Carrots (boiled)	39 + 4
6	Brown boiled rice	68 + 4	22	Milk (full fat)	39 + 3
7	Barley	28 + 2	23	Milk (skim)	37 + 4
8	Instant oat porridge	79 + 3	24	Ice cream	37 + 4
9	Rice porridge	78 + 9	25	Chick peas	28 + 9
10	Millet porridge	67 + 5	26	Soya beans	16 + 1
11	Sweet corn	52 + 5	27	Lentils	32 + 5
12	Cornflakes	81 + 6	28	Chocolate	40 + 3
13	Apple (raw)	36 + 2	29	Popcorn	65 + 5
14	Orange	43 + 3	30	Soft drinks/soda	59 + 3
15	Banana	51 + 3	31	Honey	61 + 3
16	Pineapple	59 + 8	32	Glucose	103 + 3

ANNEXURES XIII
International cut-off points for adults aged 18 years and over

Classification	**BMI score (kg/m^2)**	**Risk of co-morbidity (multiple diseases)**
Underweight	< 18.50	Low risk (but risk of other clinical problems increased)
Normal range	18.50–24.99	Average risk
Overweight	25.00–29.99	Increased risk
Obese:	≥ 30.00	High risk
Obese (class I)	30.00–34.99	Moderate risk
Obese (class II)	35.00–39.99	Severe risk
Obese (class III)	≥ 40.00	Very severe risk

ANNEXURES XIV
The International Classification of adult underweight, overweight and obesity according to BMI

Classification	**BMI(kg/m^2)**	
	Principal cut-off points	**Additional cut-off points**
Underweight	**<18.50**	**<18.50**
Severe thinness	<16.00	<16.00
Moderate thinness	16.00 - 16.99	16.00 - 16.99
Mild thinness	17.00 - 18.49	17.00 - 18.49
Normal range	**18.50 - 24.99**	**18.50 - 22.99**
		23.00 - 24.99
Overweight	**≥25.00**	**≥25.00**
Pre-obese	25.00 - 29.99	25.00 - 27.49
		27.50 - 29.99
Obese	**≥30.00**	**≥30.00**
Obese class I	30.00 - 34.99	30.00 - 32.49
		32.50 - 34.99
Obese class II	35.00 - 39.99	35.00 - 37.49
		37.50 - 39.99
Obese class III	≥40.00	≥40.00

ANNEXURES XV
Food exchange list

1. CEREAL EXCHANGES

1 Exchange= 18-21g Carbohydrate, 1-3g Protein, 85 Calories

Item	Raw (g)	Approx cooked weight (g)	Household Measure (cooked)
Rice	25(2Tbsp)	75	½ cup
Rice Flour	25(2Tbsp)	-	-
Idli	-	50	1 medium
Dosa	-	50	1 small
Wheat flour	25(3 ½ Tbsp)	-	-
Chapatti	-	25	1 medium
Sooji	25(2 Tbsp)	75	½ cup
Ragi Flour	25(3 ½ Tbsp)	75	½ cup
Bread	-	25	2 slices
Oats	25(3 ½ Tbsp)	75	½ cup
Cornflakes	25(5 Tbsp)	-	½ cup
Vermicelli	25(2 ½ Tbsp)	75	½ cup
Sago	25(3 Tbsp)	75	½ cup
Noodles	25	75	½ cup
Rice, Puffed/Flakes	-	1 cup	

(*Contd...*)

Potato	100	-	½ cup
Yam	75	-	¼ cup
Sweet potato	75	-	¼ cup
Colocasia	100	-	½ cup
Tapioca	50	-	¼ cup

Breakfast: 2 slices of bread = 1 exchange

Lunch: ½ cup cooked rice +1 chapatti = 2 exchange

Evening snacks: 1 idli = 1 exchange

Dinner: 2 chapatti = 2 exchange

2. MILK EXCHANGES

1 Exchange= 4g Carbohydrate, 1-3g Protein, 4 g Fats, 65 Calories

Item	Amount	Household Measure
Whole milk, Cow	100 ml	½ cup
Curd	100 ml	½ cup
*Skimmed milk	200 ml	1 cup
Whole milk powder	13g	3 tsp
*Skimmed milk powder	18g	5 tsp
Buffalo's milk	50 ml	¼ cup

(* fat negligible) 1 cup= 200ml, 1 teaspoon = 5 ml

3. MEAT/ CHEESE EXCHANGES

1 Meat Exchange=85 Calories, 7.5-18g Protein, 6 g Fats (CHO, Fat and Protein vary widely among the different foods in this group)

Item	Amount
Chicken	75g
Fish	75-100g
Egg	1 medium
Meat	50g
Paneer (Cottage Cheese)	35g (3 Tbsp)
Beef/Pork	75g

1. PULSE EXCHANGES

1 Exchange= 15g Carbohydrate, 6g Protein, Fats negligible

Item	Amount	Household Measure
All pulses and legumes	25g	½ cup cooked
Dals	25g	¾ cup cooked

5. VEGETABLE EXCHANGES

Commonly consumed vegetables have been grouped into two exchanges: (1) Group A and (2) Group B. both group include 100g raw vegetables or ½ cup of cooked vegetables.

GROUP A	GROUP B
30 Kcals per 100g 1 exchange=100 g or ½ cup cooked CHO upto 6%	50 to 60 Kcals per 100g 1 exchange= 100g or ½ CHO upto 6-12 %, Protein 2-3 g
Cabbage	Agathi
Celery,lettuce	Beetroot
Chow chow	Carrot
Brinjal	Drumstick leaves
Cauliflower	Turnip, coriander leaves
Mint	Onion big, mango ginger
Spinach	Field beans
White radish	Pink radish
Plantain stem	Gogu
Leafy greens- Fenugreek, Amarnath	Jackfruit tender
Cucumber	Sword, broad, cluster and double beans
Capsicum	
Drumstick	
French beans	
Green papaya	

(*Contd...*)

Khol khol	
Ladies finger	
Mushroom	
Tomato	
Pumpkin	
Gourds-Ridge, Snake, Ash and Bitter Gourd	
Green papaya	
Plantain flower	

6. FRUIT EXCHANGES

One Fruit Exchange = 40 Calories, 10g Carbohydrate

Item	Amount
Amla	4-5
Apple	1 small
Apricot	2fresh
Banana	½ small
Custard apple	1 small
Dates	2
Grapes	20
Guava	1 medium size
Grapefruit	½ small
Jackfruit	3 pcs
Jambu	10 small
Mango	1 small

(*Contd...*)

Melon	1 slice
Orange	1 average
Papaya, ripe	2"*3" slice
Peach	1 medium
Pear	1 small
Plum	2
Pineapple	1 slice
Sapota	1 small
Sweet lime	1 medium size
Strawberries	1 cup
Watermelon	1 slice (200g)

7. FAT EXCHANGES

One Exchange = Fat 10g, Carbohydrate nil, Protein nil

Item	Amount	Household Measure
Oil-any variety	10g	3tsp
Ghee/ vanaspati	10g	2 tsp
Butter	10g	2 ½ tsp
Margarine	10g	

ANNEXURES XVI

Nutrition Terminology

Allergic reaction: Immunologically induced tissue response to a foreign substance (allergen).

Alpha-linolenic acid: 18 carbon fatty acid with three double bonds; the first double bond is on the third carbon atom from the methyl end and therefore it is called n-3 fatty acid. It is abbreviated as 18: 3 n-3.

Amino acid: The fundamental building block of proteins.

Anabolism: Process by which complex materials in tissues and organs are built up from simple substances.

Antioxidants: A group of substances that prevent the damage caused by the oxidation of fatty acids and proteins by oxygen free radicals.

Balanced Diet: A diet containing all essential (macro and micro) nutrients in optimum quantities and in appropriate proportions that meet the requirements.

Beta-Carotene: A yellow - orange plant pigment which yields vitamin A by oxidation in the body.

Bifidus factor: A substance in human milk which stimulates the growth of a micro-organism (Lactobacillus bifidus) in the infants' intestine.

Body Mass Index: Body weight in relation to height. Body weight in kilograms divided by 2 height in metres .

Calorie: Unit used to indicate the energy value of foods. Quantitative requirements are expressed in terms of energy, i.e., kilocalories (Kcals). Newer unit for energy is Kjoules.

Catabolism: Process of breakdown of complex organic constituents in the body.

Cholesterol: A lipid constituent of blood and tissues derived from diet as well as from synthesis within the body.

Colostrum: The milk produced by mammals during the first few days after delivery.

CU: Consumption Unit. - One unit represents Recommended Dietary Allowance of energy for a sedentary man.

Empty calories: Term used for foods that provide only energy without any other nutrient, eg. White sugar and alcohol.

Enzymes: Biological catalysts which enhance the rate of chemical reactions in the body.

Essential fatty acids (EFA): Fatty acids like linoleic acid and alpha linolenic acid which are not made in the human body and must be supplied through the diet.

Fatty acids: Fundamental constituents of many lipids.

Fibre: Collective term for the structural parts of plant tissues which are resistant to the human digestive enzymes.

Flavonoids: Pigments widely distributed in nature in flowers, fruits and vegetables.

Food Exchange: Foods are classified into different groups for exchange. Each "exchange list" includes a number of measured foods of similar nutritive value that can be substituted inter-changeably in meal plans.

Free radicals: Highly reactive oxygen-derived species formed in the body during normal metabolic processes. They have the capacity to damage cellular components by oxidation.

High-density lipoproteins (HDL): These transport cholesterol from the extra-hepatic tissues to the liver. They are anti-atherogenic.

Hormones: Substances produced by a gland (endocrine) which are secreted directly into the blood stream to produce a specific effect on another organ.

Hyperlipidemia: An increase in the concentration of blood lipids (triglycerides and cholesterol).

Invisible fats: Fat present as an integral component of plant and animal foods such as in cereals, legumes and spices.

Lactoferrin: Minor protein of milk containing iron. Lactose intolerance: Disorder resulting from improper digestion of milk sugar called lactose, due to lack of an enzyme, lactase, in the intestinal mucosa.

Linoleic acid: Fatty acid containing 18 carbon atoms and two double bonds. The first double bond is on the sixth carbon atom from the methyl end. Therefore it is called n-6 fatty acid and is abbreviated as 18:2 n-6.

Lipids: A technical term for fats. They are important dietary constituents. The group includes triglycerides, steroids, cholesterol and other complex lipids.

Lipoproteins: Lipids are not soluble in blood; they are therefore transported as lipid and protein complexes.

Low-density lipoproteins (LDL): These transport cholesterol from the liver to tissues. High blood levels indicate that more cholesterol is being transported to tissues.

Macrocytic anaemia: Anaemia characterized by red blood cells which are larger than normal.

Macronutrients: Nutrients like carbohydrates, proteins and fats which are required in large quantities.

Metabolism: Includes catabolism and anabolism.

Microcytic anaemia: Anaemia characterized by red blood cells which are smaller than normal.

Micronutrients: Nutrients which are required in small quantities, such as vitamins and trace elements.

Monounsaturated fatty acids: Unsaturated fatty acids with one double bond. n-6 PUFA: Linoleic acid and its longer chain polyunsaturated fatty acids are collectively called n-6 PUFA. n-3 PUFA: Alpha-linolenic acid and its longer-chain polyunsaturated fatty acids are collectively called n-3 PUFA.

Phytochemicals: General name for chemicals present in plants.

Polyunsaturated fatty acids (PUFA): Unsaturated fatty acids with two or more double bonds.

Processed foods: Foods that are produced by converting raw food materials into a form suitable for eating.

Protein Energy Malnutrition (PEM): A marked dietary deficiency of both energy and protein resulting in undernutrition.

Recommended Dietary Allowances (RDA): The amounts of dietary energy and nutrients considered sufficient for maintaining good health by the people of a country.

Refined foods: Foods which have been processed to improve their appearance, colour, taste, odour or keeping quality.

Saturated fatty acids: Fatty acids containing maximum number of hydrogen atoms that each carbon atom can carry. They do not have double bonds.

Satiety: Feeling of satisfaction after food intake.

Trans-fatty acids: Are mainly produced during hydrogenation of oils; a few also occur naturally in very small quantities.

Triglycerides (Neutral fat): The major type of dietary fat and the principal form in which energy is stored in the body. A complex of fatty acids and glycerol.

Unsaturated fatty acids: Fatty acids in which there is a shortage of hydrogen atoms. The carbon atoms then become linked by double bonds. Unsaturated fatty acids are less stable than saturated fatty acids.

Visible fats: Fats and oils that can be used directly or in cooking.

Weaning foods: Foods which are used during gradual transition of the infant from breastfeeding to normal diet.

Bibliography

1. Dietary Guidelines for Indians- A Manual: 2011. National Institute of Nutrition, ICMR, Hyderabad.
2. ICMR. 2010. Nutrient Requirements and Recommended Dietary Allowances for Indians.
3. Agarwal, Anjana., and A. Udipi, Shobha.2014. Textbook of Human Nutrition. Jaypee Brothers Medical Publishers (P) Ltd. 1st Ed.
4. WHO. 2004. The International Classification of adult underweight, overweight and obesity according to BMI.
5. Seth,Veenu ., and Singh, Kalyani 2005. Diet Planning through the lifecycle, Part-: Normal Nutrition – A Practical Manual. Elite Publishing House Pvt. Ltd. 4th Ed.
6. Mahan,L.K. 2008. Krause's Food, Nutrition and Diet Therapy. W.B. Saunders co. 12th Ed.
7. Seth,Veenu ., and Singh, Kalyani 2005. Diet Planning through the lifecycle, Part-: Diet Therapy – A Practical Manual. Elite Publishing House Pvt. Ltd. 4th Ed.
8. NIN, Hyderabad. Dietary Guidelines for Indians., glossary 2011. ICMR, pg- 123-127
9. https://en.wikipedia.org/wiki/List_of_Indian_spices accessed on 5th July 2016
10. https://quizlet.com/27228425/basic-kitchen-equipment-utensils-flash-cards/ accessed on 10th June 2016.
11. http://vikaspedia.in/health/nutrition/common-nutrition-terminologies accessed on 15th June 2018.